EAT
WELL
RUN
STRONG

HELEN MORTON

First published 2021 by Compass-Publishing UK

ISBN 978-1-913713-40-9

Edited and typeset by The Book Refinery Ltd
www.thebookrefinery.com

This book is dedicated to my daughter, Holly.

One day you will be able to run faster and for longer than me.
But not yet.

Contents

INTRODUCTION

The importance of getting it right

This book is written for all the women in the world who run, or who want to start running. It's for those of you with a training plan to follow or a goal in mind, but who have no clear idea or the confidence to follow through with eating the right foods to help you achieve your running goals. It is a book for female runners of any age, speed and experience.

I am a firm believer in sharing knowledge and information, and in making people more aware of the choices they have.

This book is an evidence-based, easy-to-follow guide that debunks nutrition myths, explains the links between hormones, food and running, nails down specific training nutrition and exposes injury potential and your best nutritional recovery plan.

"You are what you eat." - Jean Anthelme Brillat-Savarin

Nutrition is about health. What you eat and drink impacts every single cell of your body. Essentially, "you are what you eat". This phrase was eloquently coined by a French lawyer, Jean Anthelme Brillat-Savarin, way back in 1826, in a book called *The Physiology of Taste*. Two hundred years on, scientific research has led to the phrase being updated. "You are what you eat, digest, absorb and utilise" is now far more commonly heard and quoted in the fast-evolving nutrition world.

The importance of getting food and drink right – and by that, I mean right for you and not slavishly following someone else's diet – is one of the foundations of good health. Once you get the other foundations right – physical activity, rest and recovery, a sense of purpose and mental strength – you'll be well on your way to a healthy, happy life.

In an ideal world, nutrition fundamentals are established first, before starting a running programme. Then, once running training is underway, nutrition practices simply need to be adjusted to factor in specific training, recovery and health needs.

In reality, thoughts of nutrition most often come into women's minds only after a few less-than-perfect races and fuelling experiences. My own running and nutrition journey has been no different, and I want to share with you everything I have theoretically and practically learned over the last twenty-four years.

How nutrition affects performance

I want to start by giving a practical example of how what you eat affects how well you run.

Think about two female runners, both taking part in their first ever 10km race. The day before the race, Runner A drinks water regularly, forgoing her usual Saturday night wine and swapping takeaway curry for a homecooked chicken risotto. She goes to bed feeling a little nervous but otherwise good. Runner B makes no changes to her typical Saturday food and drink – her regular coffee, cake, takeaway curry and wine remain in place. She goes to bed with a slight headache, feeling very full.

Race day arrives. Both runners are feeling excited yet nervous. Runner A slept well and starts the day with a large glass of water and a small bowl of porridge a couple of hours before the race is due to begin. She is ready to run. Runner B had a restless night, and her headache has gotten worse. She drinks a small glass of water alongside her usual milky coffee, shunning breakfast as she's still feeling full. She too is ready to run.

The runners line up and the start gun goes. They are off! Runners A and B are swept along with the crowd, hoping to gradually find their rhythm.

At the 3km mark, the road starts to climb – this is the first of two hills in the race. Runner A takes a breath, digs deeper and keeps going at a good pace up the hill. When the road flattens, she smiles in relief, continuing on her way. Runner B is starting to feel fatigued and looks at the hill ahead with some trepidation. Nevertheless, she continues running steadily, walking just a small section to get her breath back. When she reaches the top of the hill, she sighs heavily. *Not even halfway there yet*, she thinks.

At the 8km mark, there is an aid station handing out water bottles. Runner A takes one, thanks the marshal and continues running whilst sipping the water. Runner B slows to a walk as she approaches the station. As she is feeling extremely thirsty, she grabs two bottles of water. She drinks the first bottle quickly, keeping the second to drink during the remaining 2km.

The finish line is in sight and the race is almost over. Runner A increases her pace a little, finishing strongly with a beaming smile. She feels tired but exhilarated. Runner B has struggled through the last kilometre. Her stomach feels bloated and her legs don't seem to have enough energy in them to run properly. She crosses the line, immediately vowing "never again!"

This example may sound far-fetched, but it really does happen, illustrating how nutrition, along with a positive mindset, affects running performance. Runner A ran the race fully hydrated, rested and adequately fuelled. Runner B did not. Runner A enjoyed the 10km race, finishing strongly. Again, Runner B did not.

Learning how nutrition affects running performance, and about the best nutrition to focus on, is what this book is all about. I want you to eat well and run strong. Every one of my nutrition clients has health and performance goals they want to achieve. Using the same principles as you find in this book, I help them to get the results they desire, be that weight loss, a 5km PB (Personal Best), improved gut health, better energy levels or a combination of all of those things.

This is my expert opinion

Ever since I was a teenager watching the London Marathon on TV, I have had a passion for running. I found something about the rhythm of the activity and the camaraderie between fellow runners highly appealing. My passion for nutritious food and drink to fuel my chosen sport came much later in life, after I had realised the detrimental effect my high-sugar, alcohol and caffeine-rich diet had on my health. It was only then that I began to take an interest in how food can taste amazing and be good for our mind and body.

There are a couple of reasons why you should listen to my expert opinion. Firstly, I am a fully qualified, BANT-registered Nutritional Therapist, practising evidence-based nutrition. This means that I have the training, skills and knowledge to pass on everything I know about how nutrition supports our bodies. I work 1:1 with women who want support and guidance to change what – and how – they eat. Many of my clients are runners and some are swimmers and cyclists. Some women I work with do all three! The thing they all have in common is a desire to improve their health, as well as their sports performance. Under my expert guidance, they have all been successful in achieving their goals to a realistic timescale, whether that is losing some weight, improving digestive health or running a personal best (in some cases all three). All the nutrition work I do, including writing this book, is evidence-based, meaning there is scientific research and background reasoning behind all the nutrition practices and advice I give. We are unique beings, so we need unique nutrition advice that takes into consideration our underlying genetic and biological makeup.

The second reason why I am an expert on essential nutrition for female runners is simply because I am a female runner myself. I have lived and breathed all things running and nutrition for many years. My very first half marathon was way back in 1998. Back then, I made all the rookie mistakes – didn't do enough training, wore a poor choice of trainers, arrived too late to queue for the Portaloos and drank so much water when the race was over that I was sick on the journey home! During the last 20 years, I have been through episodes of severe PMS, had recurring injuries, given birth, gone through significant life stresses and mental health issues and undergone foot surgery, and I am now transitioning through the perimenopause. Through all these years, I have regularly run, bar 6 months after foot surgery and 8 months around pregnancy. I have run almost every distance, from 1-mile races through to ultramarathons, and many miles in between. This book is not about me and my story, though, it is about you and your nutrition, health and running.

But I want you to know that I understand and can empathise with your own running journey. I recognise the specific challenges that women face, in a way that my male running counterparts do not.

The research I have undertaken has been nothing short of thorough. Many areas of female health and running I have first-hand experience in, and for those areas where I don't, I have spoken with other experts and researched the latest scientific findings to share with you the most up-to-date, relevant information available. Nutrition science is always evolving and changing, as we find out more about how food and drink affects our bodies and exercise potential. All the information given in this book is correct at the time of going to press. In fifty years, who knows what will have changed?

There's lots of misunderstandings out there

It's true that there is a lot of misunderstood and badly researched information out there. At best, misleading articles are confusing; at worst, they are dangerous. A quick search of nutrition and running-related information returns thousands of results. A lot of it comes from old wives' tales or extreme diets that have no sound scientific evidence behind them. I am not saying that all this type of information is unproven. However, there is a lot of unsubstantiated nonsense around, so I encourage you to think carefully about what you read and the source of the information.

One of the most dangerous things about social media and the world wide web is the number of self-proclaimed health 'experts' touting certain foods, diets and ways of eating as miracle cures for any number of things. We'd all like to believe that there is one simple fix for our health concerns and achieving a better running performance, but you must think carefully before following someone else's diet. What works for one person will not necessarily work for you. Also, bear in mind that you do not really know what is going on behind the scenes of a social media post. A handful of pictures do not tell a person's whole health and fitness story.

What you will learn from this book

I will cover everything you need to know about nutrition for female runners. Think of it as a journey, similar to the one you go on from when you first hear about a race you want to do, to crossing the finish line and getting your coveted medal placed around your neck. Believe me, I can make anything related to running!

Section 1 – These are the building blocks of nutrition, the starting point and basis for eating well and running strong.

Chapter 1 debunks some of the myths surrounding female running nutrition. Everything from the obsession with sports drinks, to the myth of needing to eat meat as a protein source, to women being treated the same as men when we are blatantly different.

Chapter 2 goes through nutrition basics. It includes all the important things you need to know about carbohydrates, dietary fat and protein, plus sugar, alcohol and hydration. This chapter is a combination of practical advice and scientific research.

Chapter 3 is much more specific to female runners, focusing on some of the different types of hormonal challenges we may face over the course of our lifetime.

Chapter 4 focuses on running to lose weight. Dr Eve Pearce, Scientific Officer at myDNAhealth, the award-winning nutritional genomics and epigenetics company, discusses the role of genetics in relation to running and weight loss.

Chapter 5 goes into detail about the most common mental health issues female runners contend with, and the nutritional strategies to support us during these periods.

Section 2 – Training nutrition. In Chapters 6, 7 and 8, I provide specific advice and fuelling requirements tailored to different distances and types of training, starting from building up to consistent 5km running, through to ultramarathon events.

Section 3 – After care, the often neglected running and wellbeing fundamentals.

Chapter 9 goes into detail concerning how what you eat and drink can impact the risk of sustaining injuries, and I share practical nutrition advice on essential recovery after running.

Chapter 10 highlights the importance of sleep for optimal health and a strong running performance, including the nutritional strategies that help promote restful slumber, and those that do not.

Chapter 11 is written by Clare Flaxen, a Cognitive Behavioural Therapist, and shows you how to create lasting change with nutrition and running, and make your goals a reality. There are also links to downloadable PDFs where you can fill out answers to specific questions/goals.

Throughout this book, you will find information on sources of nutrients, as well as greyed out boxes designed to make the reading experience more practical and enjoyable.

There are a few recipes within the book, but my main aim is to guide you towards the foods that suit you, leaving you to decide how best to incorporate them into your diet. However, as many female runners do want some guidance on the meals and snacks that could be adapted to their individual needs, by the end of 2022, I will have published a companion recipe book designed to help you achieve your running goals.

Whatever level of runner you are and for however long you have been pounding the streets, I suggest that you follow this book through from beginning to end. There may well be chapters that are not so applicable to you right now, but hopefully you will gain some knowledge or understanding from each section that you can either put into practice yourself or pass onto another runner. Let's get you started.

SECTION 1

BUILDING
BLOCKS

This first section starts by debunking the common running nutrition myths, before moving onto practical advice about the nutrition basics that female runners need to know. Then it's time to delve deeper, into nutrition for hormone balance, weight management and mental health.

CHAPTER 1

DEBUNKING MYTHS

This first chapter is necessary, as it gets rid of several of the most common misconceptions around nutrition and running. These are things you may have heard about, and possibly already unsuccessfully tried yourself. These types of myths often lead women like you to make the wrong nutritional choices. Some of them are so embedded in running lore that surely they must be true, right? I am here to tell you that no, they are not.

Carb loading

If you are already a marathon runner then amazing! What an awesome achievement. During your training, you will more than likely have heard the term 'carb loading', perhaps from articles in popular running magazines, and on websites and social media shares. Maybe you have also chatted with other runners about carb loading.

Most information for runners gives the impression that in order to run a good, strong race, you must eat copious quantities of carbohydrate-rich foods, such as bread and pasta. I hold my hands up. I got caught by this nutrition myth from 2002 to 2006, the years when my running distances first increased, culminating in me taking part in the London Marathon, which was my first ever marathon distance. The night before the race, I remember searching for a restaurant where I could order a large bowl of pasta. In the morning, I felt relieved to find a café that served porridge and honey, so my high-carb breakfast routine was not broken. The question is, did these high-carb meals benefit my running? Dinner certainly did not. I ended the day feeling overly full and uncomfortable, which meant I slept ridiculously badly. Though, let's be honest, nerves also played a part in getting such little sleep. I arrived at the start feeling bloated and uncomfortable, a far cry from the smiling, energetic vision I had in mind. Despite training with jelly sweets and isotonic sports drinks, because back then that was the only fuelling strategy I knew about, all my plans went out of the window on marathon day and fuelling during the race was minimal. Unsurprisingly, by mile 19, I had crashed. Suffice to say, all those carbs I ate in the 24 hours before the marathon did not help with running anywhere near a perfect marathon. (Though I admit I still loved every minute!)

"Eat the right type of carbs, in the right quantities, at the right time." - Helen Morton

For those of you unfamiliar with the term 'carb loading' and wondering what on earth I am talking about, let me explain. This is about maximising the body's glycogen (energy) stores through consuming a high-carbohydrate diet, supposedly allowing you to run for longer before needing to top up with more carbohydrates. It is a strategy commonly used by endurance athletes, whether they are runners, cyclists or triathletes. Why carbohydrates? Because carbs are your body's main energy source. The carbohydrates you eat are broken down into sugars (glucose), which are stored in your muscles and liver in the form of glycogen, ready to be utilised by the body as you run. In Chapter 2, I go into much more detail about carbohydrate foods, and why, as runners, you do need to be eating some carbs, but the right type in the right quantities at the right time.

How carb loading began

The strategy of carb loading was initially born in the 1960s, from lab studies in Scandinavia, when researchers first experimented with depleting their muscles of glycogen by restricting their carbohydrate intake and exercising intensely, followed by a four-day carbohydrate binge. These runners took needle biopsies of their leg muscles to see how glycogen stores were altered, concluding that this protocol maximised pre-exercise muscle glycogen. In other words, loading up on carbs gave their leg muscles maximum stored energy. Top British runner Ron Hill became an ambassador for carb loading after his spectacular 1969 marathon win at the European Athletics Championships, where he overtook the front runner with one kilometre to go, an act he put down to not slowing down in the same way as his competitor. Ron attributed his racing success to the high-carb diet he had been following. Encouraged by his win, aspiring competitive runners followed suit by changing their own diets pre-race, and so carb-loading for runners started to take off.

The original 1960s carb loading studies were followed by further research in the 1980s. These later studies excluded the initial glycogen depletion phase, focusing instead on increased carbohydrate intake and decreased training for the three days before an endurance event. Researchers found that a diet of 70 per cent carbohydrates, from bread, pasta, rice and potatoes, combined with minimal training for 72 hours, had the effect of maximising glycogen levels in participants' muscles and liver. What these lab studies failed to test, however, was the athletes' actual running performance during a marathon event, having followed the diet and training protocols. Invasive muscle biopsies were taken but no running was done. Lab studies are all well and good, but real-life research and analysis is arguably more important. By that I mean actual running performance rather than what tests and blood work show. As I'll explain, it is best to take research studies into consideration rather than following them to the letter.

The problems

I think that one of the problems with the term 'carb loading' is that the word 'loading' implies excess. Being told to eat any amount of bread, potatoes and pasta you like before a long run sounds great, right? We all like to cling to beliefs that appear simple and enjoyable, but sadly, eating carbohydrates excessively in the hope of running longer, stronger and faster is a myth. Though admittedly, as I have explained, it's a myth born out of solid scientific research. However, like a lot of nutrition research, real-life practical implementation for the thousands of regular runners who run long distances has been lost. More recent research has shown that the cycle of depleting and loading muscle glycogen is not always helpful, or indeed necessary. The most successful endurance runners are less likely to follow a strict carb depletion/load plan and are more likely to tailor their carbohydrate intake to the training they are doing. This is nothing excessive, they are simply fuelling for the work required.

Returning briefly to research, in one study on endurance cyclists, men and women were asked to increase their carbohydrate intake before a cycle test. The male cyclists significantly improved performance time and muscle glycogen stores, yet the female cyclists didn't. When the participants' diets were analysed, it was found that the male athletes consumed an average of 8.2g per kg of body weight of carbohydrate, while on average, the women consumed 6.4g per kg of body weight. The men took on more carbohydrates than the women. Several studies suggest that there is a "carbohydrate loading threshold" of 8–10g per kg of body weight that is necessary to achieve the ergogenic benefits of carb loading, indicating that in this instance, the female athletes may not have taken on enough carbohydrates for performance benefits. Carbohydrate intake relative to lean body mass is an important consideration, rather than intake relative to overall body weight. This is important for you to know, as it is widely accepted that in general, women have greater body fat and less fat-free mass than men.

Female runners are not men

When it comes to running, men and women are different, and that is a good thing! As far as I'm concerned, you are the superior sex, but there is no getting away from the fact that women tend to have a smaller liver and muscles compared with their male counterparts. This limits your glycogen storage capacity. If you are a well-trained female runner, you may be able to store sufficient glycogen to fuel up to potentially 20 miles of running, but it's highly unlikely that this will be enough for the whole marathon distance. No matter how many bowls of pasta or porridge you eat in the 48 hours before running a marathon, your glycogen storage capacity will remain unchanged. Any extra carbohydrate consumed will be stored as fat, of which, sadly, there is an almost unlimited storage capacity.

Another thing to consider is that emerging evidence indicates glycogen storage does not occur in the same manner for male and female athletes. This is due to hormones. Yep, your pesky essential hormones are at play again! It appears that one of the steroid hormones secreted by female ovaries plays an important role in the gender differences seen in carbohydrate metabolism and storage. Where you are in your menstrual cycle has been shown to have a direct impact on glycogen storage, and, therefore, how your body handles the carbohydrate foods you eat before a long run or race. Read onto Chapter 3 for more on female hormones and running performance.

Most research is done on men and elite runners

Yes, you read that right. Most research studies related to how humans respond to activity and nutrition stimulus are done using male subjects, most commonly higher performing male athletes. Women like you have had to rely on nutrition advice, training plans and injury protocols based on research on men – men who have many biological differences.

For starters, as I have already touched upon, in general, men have a greater body mass than women. This means that their caloric and macronutrient (that's protein, fat and carbohydrates) requirements are greater than they are for women. Vitamin and mineral needs for men and women are also different. Females tend to require higher levels, especially iron and magnesium. This is partly due to your menstrual cycle, which I will talk about more in Chapter 3. It's also partly because research shows that as we age, we metabolise magnesium to a lesser extent, meaning we need to consume more to get the same effect as we did in our younger years. These same changes in magnesium metabolism do not appear to occur in men as they grow older. Lucky them! These are just two examples of how women respond differently to the same nutrition, highlighting the flaws in female runners following research studies based solely on male athletes.

Another example of distorted information surrounds calcium needs. There is evidence that a high consumption of the mineral may be harmful to men in terms of prostate health, and there is little evidence that dietary calcium is protective for them in the development of osteoporosis. Meanwhile, the opposite is true for women. A higher calcium intake, in conjunction with magnesium and vitamin D, can go some way to protecting you from the bone disease. If someone writes an article or paper based solely on male participant research studies, the information given about calcium needs may be skewed, most likely indicating a lower amount than you need. At best, this can leave you confused, and at worst deficient in calcium and at greater risk of injury and poor bone health. In a similar way, scientific studies have found gender gaps in the way people absorb and benefit from omega-3 fatty acids.

Why are women left out?

So, why are more research studies done on men than women? Primarily, I believe, it is because men are generally the ones making the decisions and conducting the research. It is a simple fact that there are more men than women in the world of scientific research, and the decision makers tend to choose the easier option – male participants. Unless, of course, it's a study that specifically requires women.

The reasoning behind a large majority of sports science studies using solely male participants comes down to two main factors: time and money. Studying women's responses to nutritional interventions can take longer and cost more. Now throw in the added factor that in the past more men than women have participated in running events and sport, giving scientists a greater number of male subjects to choose from. Thankfully, that is slowly starting to change, as more women like you start running.

A multitude of research studies are conducted with high performing and elite runners. Why them and not regular club or recreational runners? Primarily, elite athletes can be easier to study because they are the sports people with access to high-tech gyms and equipment. They are also frequently part of large training groups, are consistent with training and will have regular tests taken, their times assessed and their diets controlled, making them, as a group, more straightforward to monitor than athletes who train on their own.

This is all understandable, but the question is, can the analysis of the response of high-performing athletes to training and nutrition be turned into something appropriate and useful for female recreational runners like you and me? Training loads, life loads, body shape and many other factors differ between elite and recreational runners. I can think of no similarities, other than we all run, between the group of women I usually train with and the young elite runners racing the London Marathon. Of course, elite runners are humans just like the rest of us, even if they seem a world apart!

Research studies extrapolate, which means, for instance, they can estimate how a nutritional intervention will affect the general population based on a small number of research subjects. If the subjects have sufficient similarities with regular runners then estimations can be accurate and applicable. If, however, research participants are Kenyan male elite runners in their 20s, using data on how they reacted to a certain nutritional intervention may not always result in the most accurate estimation of how an English, post-menopausal, slightly overweight female runner lacing up her trainers for the first time in years will respond. Some studies do consider differences in people, but not all of them, so I think it is important to be aware of this. In the best case scenario, you could be persuaded to consume a food that is ineffective and does nothing to support your health or running. In the worst case, unlikely as it is, you could be unknowingly doing yourself harm.

One thing I wondered when writing this chapter is why there aren't more studies done on female non-elite runners. Sadly, the answer is mainly because of the two factors mentioned earlier: time and money

Studying a group of female athletes with fluctuating hormones and physiological variability is simply more expensive and takes longer. This is because female hormones affect several parameters, such as hydration and temperature regulation, metabolism of macro and micronutrients and levels of fatigue. Some decision makers shy away from the complexity and length of time it takes to design and analyse such data from women.

Menstruation is another reason why women are shunned in research studies. The stage of the monthly cycle a woman is in needs to be considered, which, as mentioned above, increases complexity and, therefore, costs. And with budgets often already limited, sadly, some studies on female athletes never get off the ground.

Light at the end of the tunnel

Thankfully, the number of nutrition studies on female athletes is starting to slowly change, with more female-based research being undertaken. But there is still a long way to go. An evaluation of more than 1,300 exercise medicine studies published between 2011 and 2013 found that just 39 per cent of study subjects were women. In a follow-up review of 188 studies published in early 2015, women accounted for 42 per cent of study participants. In the field of sports science, the figures are even lower; just 3 per cent of participants were found to be women. I do wonder how this can be. Us women make up around half of the population, yet scientific studies are based mainly on men. The issue is that if sweeping assumptions are made, how good is the data and advice that comes out of these studies? With the increasing appreciation by all levels of runners that women experience aspects of training, recovery and injury differently to men and, therefore, benefit from sex-specific research and guidelines, I passionately believe that things needs to change.

Despite common misinformation, I am in no way saying that every running magazine or internet article you read should be disregarded under the assumption that it was written for men by men and is, therefore, not applicable to you. Or that research was done purely with elite athletes so cannot be relevant to us slower runners. What I am saying is to bear in mind that the advice given may not be suitable for your own needs. Consider it and be sensible in your response, using your own experiences and situation to make informed decisions. If needed, talk to nutrition professionals like me. Do not slavishly follow advice to eat specific quantities or types of food if that does not feel right to you. As I will explain further, the idea of one type of nutrition fitting all is a myth.

Couch to 5k overeating

This section is for those of you embarking on your running journey, perhaps using the ever-popular Couch to 5k programme.

I believe we all have an inbuilt desire to reward ourselves after having done something we feel is hard work, even if that's something we also kind of enjoy. When you first start out running, or are returning to running after an injury, it feels hard. Extremely hard. Even keeping going for 10 minutes of running/walking can feel tough. And when you do something challenging or difficult, your brain is hardwired to want a pleasure reward afterwards. In an ideal world, I'd like every female runner to do it for enjoyment rather than punishment or reward. Running is so freeing and meditative; it should be a pleasure not a chore. (Yes, there will be days when it feels tough. On these days, I recommend looking to the skies, to your surroundings, to the feel of your body and the joy of movement.)

Pleasurable rewards after completing your run could include a relaxing bubble bath, a Netflix binge or simply a happy dance in the kitchen. But I get it, these things do not always cut it. Sometimes you want something more indulgent. You want food! For many women, exercise is a way of burning off calories and purging their overindulgence, even though that is an outdated practice because your body just does not work like that. Conversely, you may be a woman who views exercise simply as a pass to eat more of what you fancy. Our relationship with food can be complicated, often stemming from childhood learned behaviours, and when exercise is thrown into the mix, rewards and rules become even more intertwined. The psychology of eating and food choice is a fascinating topic, elements of which you will find dotted around this book, especially in Chapter 5 on mental health.

Running for weight loss

Some women start a Couch to 5k programme at the same time as embarking on a strict diet to try and shed some weight. There is a mistaken belief that by increasing exercise duration (how long for) and intensity (how hard/fast) while reducing your calorie intake, the pounds will automatically drop off. Unfortunately, weight loss is not so simple. Your body is a clever thing. It has an inbuilt survival mechanism and is always trying to make sure we do not starve. Once your body senses that starvation is occurring, when long-term food intake is deficient in nutrients or energy, it shifts into survival mode, holding onto every little bit of energy it can. Body weight does not decrease, rather the opposite often occurs, as your body stores food for emergency purposes.

A note on technology. In recent years, fitness trackers and apps have become a popular way to track calorie intake and expenditure from food consumed and exercise taken. However, when it comes to energy burned during physical activity, many studies have shown most fitness trackers to be misleading. Their accuracy in measuring calorie expenditure varies widely. Research found that devices tended to slightly underestimate energy expenditure, leading to concerns that some people may overdo exercise, increasing stress on their cardiovascular system and raising injury risk. On the other hand, inaccuracy through these gadgets overestimating energy expenditure leads to the opposite problem, giving a false impression of your energy requirements. By regularly consuming more food than your body requires, you can easily gain weight, which is the opposite of what so many women starting off on their 5km running journey want.

Appetite and hunger

A common thing I hear from many of my nutrition clients and fellow runners is that they feel hungry straight after running. This may well feel true for you, however, there is no scientific evidence, on either men or women, to support this phenomenon. In fact, it's quite the opposite. Several studies have shown that appetite tends to be supressed after undertaking physical activity. One large study of endurance runners (mainly men, some women) found participants' appetite decreased after training, which is thought to be caused by alterations in body temperature.

Nothing in sports science is simple, though. Physical activity and its impact on appetite has many factors, including fitness level, body fat percentage and your ability to recognise hunger cues. Hormones also play a vital role. Exercise is known to decrease levels of the appetite-stimulating hormone ghrelin while increasing levels of the appetite-suppressing hormone leptin. However, it seems that exercise's hunger-suppressing effects do not happen for everyone in quite the same way. Research shows that leptin hormones respond differently in obese women compared with lean ones, though how and why that is remains unclear.

Genetics also play a role, with nutrition being one of the cornerstones to how we respond to different foods and training. In Chapter 4, Dr Eve Pearce, Scientific Officer for myDNAhealth, shares everything you need to know about genetics, lifestyle and nutrition.

For women embarking on a running journey with Couch to 5k or another beginner running programme, the intensity of your exercise will play a significant role in your appetite. Higher-intensity workouts, such as speed sessions, interval training or racing, tend to temporarily suppress appetite. This is because during intense exercise, blood supply is redirected to the important jobs performed by your heart, muscles and brain, leaving less for the digestive system, hence appetite suppression. Low and moderate-intensity exercise, such as walking and jogging, do not have the same effect on your blood supply and may slightly increase your appetite. This is something to watch out for as you start running and walking more often.

"Eat what you need for the activity you do." - Helen Morton

One of the most important things when embarking on a running and weight-loss programme is balance. One mantra many sports nutritionists live by is, *"fuel for the work required"*. Section 2 of this book covers training nutrition, giving specific guidance on running distances from 5km upwards. Doing shorter, lower intensity runs a couple of times a week requires no real increase in food consumption, particularly if you are looking to lose some weight. Whether a 5km run takes you 40 minutes or half that, cakes and indulgent coffees afterwards are not the best reward in terms of weight loss or health. Occasionally they're fine, but not every single time you run. Keep those kinds of food and drink as an irregular treat, not a regular weekly reward. I am guessing there was a reason behind you taking up running, a 'why' that is in your head every time you lace up your trainers. Keep your goals and your overarching purpose in mind after running as well as before.

Lucozade Sport – the sports drink myth

OK, hands up if you've ever been caught out by this myth at some point, the one telling you that if a running event, like most marathons, is sponsored by a particular brand of sports drink, you should be consuming it during each training run and on the race day itself. Back in 2006, I was well and truly caught by this marketing trap and did all of my London Marathon training fuelled by sickly sweet sports drinks that I did not enjoy. This was simply because that's what the London Marathon magazine (which you are sent if you are successful in getting a ballot place) told me to do, and I did not think to question the all-knowing London Marathon team.

I can tell you here and now that you do not need to consume sports drinks to successfully run a marathon. All the promo material may shout otherwise, but please ignore it. The fact is, big running events like the London Marathon are commercial ventures and sponsorship is all about money, with less interest in the health and performance of the participants. If the sports drink in question is one you happen to enjoy and run well on, then by all means keep drinking it, but if you do not like the taste and the drink upsets your stomach please, please avoid it. Nobody is going to pull you from an event for choosing a different drink.

Types of sports drinks

There are three types of sports drink, each containing various levels of fluid, electrolytes and carbohydrates. These are hypotonic, isotonic and hypertonic. Commercial sports drinks, such as the ones given out during races, are designed to supplement training. These are isotonic drinks, containing similar concentrations of sugar and salt as you find in your body. They are meant to quickly replace the fluids you lose during exercise and replenish essential carbohydrates, which come in the form of glucose, maltodextrin and/or fructose. This, by the way, can be the cause of stomach issues. High carbohydrate drinks upset digestive function in many runners, causing loose stools, nausea or a heavy feeling in the tummy, sometimes all three. If you have ever had the misfortune of feeling like this, you will know what I am talking about.

GI distress

Gastrointestinal (GI) distress in runners is common, especially in marathon runners, as they are more likely to take on board sports drinks or energy gels during training and racing. Back in 1988, almost a quarter of the runners who had just finished the Belfast City Marathon were questioned on various GI problems they had encountered during training. A massive 83 per cent of them reported experiencing problems at least occasionally during training, with diarrhoea and urgent bowel movements being the most common. Women and younger runners seem more susceptible to GI issues, although it isn't clear exactly why this is. Causes are multifactorial, but there's no doubt that the food you eat before and during running plays a role.

Downsides of sports drinks

The main issue with sports drinks is that the big brands, like Lucozade and Powerade, generally produce drinks that are not healthful because they contain excessive quantities of sugar, artificial sweeteners, colourings, preservatives and other nasties. Although advertising may imply otherwise, for example, Lucozade launched a campaign in 2014 promoting the drink as 'fuel to rule', there is a lack of evidence that these types of drinks have any benefits. On the contrary, recent studies report damage to heart health and the liver when consuming sports drinks excessively.

Moreover, the sugar content tends to be extremely high in these drinks, up to 20g in a 500ml bottle, and the types of sugar are far from natural. For example, orange Lucozade Sport contains glucose syrup and two different types of artificial sweeteners. Preservatives are added, which admittedly have their uses, but your body sees them as toxins, which your liver needs to process and get rid of. Plus, Lucozade Sport contains acidity regulators, added colours, flavours and food dyes. None of these ingredients are beneficial for runners.

Sugar

An additional issue with sugars in sports drinks is the impact they have on your teeth. Now, your pearly whites may be the last thing on your mind when training for a race, but there are many incidences of tooth decay in athletes, all attributed to drinks and gels. One recent study found that 49 per cent of top-performing athletes have untreated tooth decay, while 32 per cent of the athletes studied reported their oral health had a negative impact on their training and performance. It is thought that more than 85 per cent of athletes regularly consume sports drinks, up to 60 per cent eat energy bars and 70 per cent regularly use energy gels, all of which are known to damage teeth. The sugars in these products increase your chance of developing tooth decay, while the acidity raises the risk of enamel erosion. By using sports drinks too often, you could be causing your teeth harm without even realising it.

Sports drinks generally have little nutritional value, though it must be said that some have added vitamins and minerals. For example, small quantities of vitamin B6, B12, niacin and pantothenic acid are added to orange Lucozade Sport. But isn't it better to get all the vitamins you need through whole, natural foods?

Do you need to refuel?

Think back to the previous section on Couch to 5k overeating. The marketing myth of sports drinks does not just relate to marathon running, there seems to be a common belief that any exercise we do, whether that is working out in the gym or running outside, needs to be accompanied by a sugary sports drink. This just isn't the case. Some longer types of exercise do need more careful consideration around hydration and fuelling, but a 40-minute gym or run session generally requires you to drink no more than good old plain water. This is perfectly adequate, and it comes from the tap without added calories, sugars or processed nasties.

Finally, do not give up hope. Sports nutrition is a booming industry and new companies are popping up all the time with more natural products. If you fancied, you could always save a few pounds per bottle and make your own simple sports drink using only natural ingredients.

One way of eating

Humans are unique beings. Just look at all the runners milling around at the start of a race or running through your local park on a Saturday morning. You'll see all sorts of shapes and sizes, not to mention different ages, speeds and running forms

---

Homemade isotonic sports drink:

» 2 cups filtered water
» 2 cups coconut water
» 2 tbsp freshly squeezed lemon juice
» 1 tbsp honey
» ¼ tsp Himalayan pink salt

Simply mix together and drink as required.

"One size does not fit all." - Frank Zappa

When it comes to nutrition, there is no one-size-fits-all approach. It is too simplistic to expect there to be one single way of eating that works for every single woman who runs. We all have foods that suit us and those that do not. Some of us have food allergies or intolerances, others may feel able to eat any type of food going but have a low tolerance for caffeine. Generic nutrition guidance, like aiming to eat a minimum of five fruit and veg a day, is a brilliant start, especially if your diet is less than ideal to begin with. However, specific advice is much more useful and powerful for you and your unique goals.

A large project has been undertaken jointly by King's College London and Massachusetts General Hospital, looking at nutrition data from over 1,000 adults in the UK and US, 60 per cent of whom were twins. Results from the study revealed wide variations in the blood glucose responses of participants consuming the same meals. This was partly, but not fully, explained by genetic differences. The project found that identical twins sharing the same genes and some of the same environmental factors frequently responded differently to the same meal. Researchers believe that gut microbiome variations may account for some of these different responses. The identical twins taking part in the project were found to share just 37 per cent of their gut bacteria. This wasn't significantly different to the 35 per cent of gut bacteria shared between two unrelated participants. This study also revealed large differences in responses to the same meal, depending on the time of day it was eaten.

Even just this one large-scale project shows that your gut microbiome, meal timings, genetics and exercise levels and intensity can result in different responses. One type of food or meal affects people differently at different times. This dispels the myth of one rule for all when it comes to nutrition.

Macronutrient ratios

One misconception of nutrition for runners is that we should all be eating the same ratio of macronutrients – that is carbohydrates, protein and dietary fats – and quantities of micronutrients, vitamins and minerals. As far as I'm concerned, this is utter nonsense. Rather, you need to be eating the correct ratios and quantities of nutrients that are right for you, your training, your biochemical imbalances, your lifestyle and your genetics.

It's foolish to expect all runners, and people in general, to be eating the same quantity and variety of food every day.

Imagine a 55-year-old, 12 stone, 5'10" 5km runner, compared with a 25-year-old, 8 stone, 5' 2" half-marathon runner. They're at different stages of their life, with different hormones, weights, training goals, life loads and stresses. You get the picture – different people have different nutritional needs. The younger, faster runner may well thrive on a higher carbohydrate diet; it is less likely that the older runner will do so to the same extent. Conversely, the older runner may be on long-term medication to manage chronic health conditions, necessitating them to avoid certain foods; the younger runner may need those same foods as part of their healthy, balanced, running-performance diet.

In Chapter 6, I talk in detail about training nutrition, specifically regarding how running distance and intensity requires different strategies. Think about it. Would you need the same diet to fuel you through a 40-mile-a-week marathon training schedule and a 5-mile-a-week general fitness plan? Not likely. Marathon training requires more attention to nutrition and a different balance of macronutrients than shorter training distances do.

The appeal

I totally get that an off-the-shelf meal plan or nutrition manual may seem appealing, because we all want an easier life. Wouldn't it be great to follow one meal plan that solves all our problems and the concerns of what to eat and when, with a list of foods that we stick to every week of every year? Sadly, this approach fails to consider several significant things: lifestyle, medical history, budget, time availability and food preferences, amongst others.

Meal plans are not successful if the recipes are too time-consuming, expensive, challenging, unsuitable for health issues or simply do not appeal. I found that out early on in my nutrition career. Giving my clients a food plan to follow with meals based around foods they don't like or have the time to cook is not useful or successful. If you aren't careful, what starts off as a plan to make your life simpler and easier can swiftly transform into a headache and just another thing to do and sort out. And the plan will eventually be discarded in favour of old (and probably less healthy) nutritional habits.

Personalised is best

A personalised, individual approach to nutrition provides better long-term health benefits than a prescriptive, one-size-fits-all plan. It looks under the surface, digs deep and uncovers imbalances that target and address what is really going on with an individual.

I qualified as a Nutritional Therapy practitioner in 2015, after studying with the Institute for Optimum Nutrition for 4 years.

Nutritional therapy is the application of nutrition science in the promotion of health, peak performance and individual care. I use a wide range of tools to assess and identify potential nutritional imbalances and understand how these may contribute to an individual's symptoms and health concerns. It's like having a complex puzzle to solve, and I love it!

Protein only comes from animal sources

According to The Vegan Society, in 2019, there were 600,000 vegans in Great Britain alone, a fourfold increase from the 150,000 vegans in 2014. This is undoubtedly why non-meat sources of protein have become such a popular topic of conversation in the sporting world. More and more runners are trying out plant-based diets, frequently for the health benefits and sometimes for ethical reasons, too.

Chapter 2 delves into protein in more detail, what it is and why it is so essential for female runners, but for now, let's keep things clear and simple: protein is a component of both animal and plant foods. It is perfectly possible to consume sufficient protein from a solely plant-based diet. I am not saying that this kind of diet suits everyone, or indeed that a meat-based diet does (refer to the previous section on one type of nutrition not fitting all). I am simply exposing the myth that protein only comes from animal sources.

For a long time, the sporting world has held concerns over whether vegan and vegetarian diets are sufficient to support the performance goals and nutritional requirements of athletes. Speculation has been rife that to perform at our highest level, consuming animal products is necessary.

History of protein consumption

Protein is vital for our survival, but we don't actually need to consume as much of it as previously thought. In the Western world, on average, we eat more than we need. The myth that we should be eating more dates back to the early 20th century, when scientists believed it was the key to wiping out child malnutrition in developing countries. In the 1960s, the protein myth continued when a United Nations report was published identifying worldwide protein deficiency. The report called for a 'global strategy to avert the impending protein crisis', and so international aid focusing on addressing the so-called 'protein gap' was born. Projects such as the subsidised production of dried milk powder to provide high-quality protein for the world's poor were launched.

Even so, reports about increasing protein consumption were not wholly accepted by scientists. Conflicting reports in the 1950s and 1960s found that higher protein diets made no more of a difference to weight gain than other types of food intake. Then in 1969, researchers concluded that almost all staple foods contain sufficient protein for our needs. Yet still the animal-based high protein diet myth remains.

As I have already said, it is perfectly possible to consume sufficient protein to run at the best of your ability from a solely plant-based diet. There is no avoiding the fact that plant foods, on the whole, contain less protein than animal foods, but with some thought and planning you can certainly get what your body needs (20g of protein is a sensible portion size at main meals for most female runners).

Examples of foods supplying 20g of protein:

- » 25g whey protein powder
- » 60g chicken or turkey breast
- » 70g beef fillet steak
- » 100g white fish
- » 3 whole eggs
- » 417g natural yoghurt
- » 33g spirulina powder
- » 100g cashews
- » 5 tbsp peanut butter
- » 120g chia seeds
- » 150g oats

» 250g tofu
» 400g baked beans
» 400g peas
» 500g broccoli

As you can see from the list above, greater quantities of plant foods need to be consumed to hit the 20g of protein mark. For example, a whole pack of tofu is equivalent to eating a third of a chicken breast. Once you know what you are aiming for you can plan around that.

Plant-based athletes

On a positive note, when it comes to 'plant-based athletes' there are plenty of examples of high-profile female sportswomen who don't eat meat and have succeeded in their chosen field. These include the 7-times Grand Slam winner, Venus Williams, who changed her diet after being diagnosed with the autoimmune disease Sjogren's syndrome, which can cause joint pain. In the running community, Catra Corbett, a colourful, tattooed American super ultramarathon runner consumes a solely plant-based diet. She has completed more than 250 ultramarathons, including more than a hundred 100-mile races. That is a lot of running! Catra has been quoted as saying that "eating clean and being vegan helps me with recovery and keeps me healthy". Fiona Oakes, another world-renowned ultra-endurance athlete also reportedly follows a plant-based diet, with great success. Fiona holds the record for being the fastest woman to complete the ice marathon in Antarctica, an amazing achievement that most of us can only dream about. So, if plant-based eating works for these successful female athletes, then perhaps it could work for some regular runners, too.

What this all means

One thing I think is important for female runners to bear in mind when choosing to eat less meat and more plant foods is under fuelling, which is when you don't eat enough to fuel the training you do. Studies show that female vegan athletes are more likely than meat eaters to do this. Not just in terms of the quantity of food and energy, but also by consuming insufficient dietary fat, iron, vitamin B12 and calcium. Under fuelling can lead to reduced performance, recurrent injuries, mood swings and long-term health issues. Head to Chapter 5 for more on the dangers of this.

Whatever the studies indicate, with thought and planning, female runners can consume sufficient protein, run strongly and remain healthy on a solely-plant based diet.

CHAPTER 2

NUTRITION BASICS

What the reader needs to know

I would like to take this opportunity to reiterate what I explained right at the beginning of this book. The food and drink you choose to consume on a regular basis make up one of the fundamental foundations of strong, healthy running. Some foods provide all the energy you need to run well, while others make you feel sluggish and slow. Sometimes, it's what is missing in your diet that stops you from running as far or as fast as you would like.

This chapter is arguably the most important one of the entire book, as it covers all the nutrition basics you need to know, whatever stage of your running journey and life you are currently at.

These are the essentials of nutrition that every female runner needs to know, from the most useful types of carbohydrates and proteins for runners, to why dietary fat really is necessary for women (spoiler, the type of fat you regularly eat is important), plus the significant role that drinks play in running performance.

> If you implement my advice, I guarantee you'll be running stronger in no time at all.

Carbohydrates, proteins, fats

These are the three macronutrients, and they are foods your body demands in large quantities, whether you are a runner or not. Each has their own function and reason for being a requirement for women. The finer details concerning how much is best to eat, when and the different types of these essential foods is the extra bit to understand.

As already mentioned, in the athletic world, the ideal quantities and ratios of each macronutrient has long been discussed and argued over, as I expect they will be for years to come. When I first started learning about nutrition, I was taught 65/15/20 as the 'ideal' for all runners (65 per cent of calories from carbohydrates, 15 per cent from proteins, 20 per cent from fats), regardless of age, gender or build. This is ludicrous. How can one single way of eating be right for me in my 20s, when I weighed a tiny 46kg (7st2lb), ran 35 miles a week and did no other exercise AND me now, heading towards 50, weighing a good 4kg (6lb) more, and running 20 miles a week but doing regular strength training and other exercise? I don't believe it can.

Thankfully, nowadays, there are a whole range of 'ideals' depending on age, individual biochemistry, genetics, training status and overarching goals. It comes down to one thing. Individuality. The things that make you *you* and me *me*.

All the 'one-size-fits-all' macronutrient ratios are great as a starting point, but they are not something to stick to resolutely. What you really need is to find the equilibrium that works for you, at any moment in time.

Carbohydrates

You have already read about carbohydrates in Chapter 1, when I debunked the myth of carb loading and explained why eating all the pasta in sight is highly unlikely to make you a faster, stronger runner.

This section of the book delves deeper into everything you need to know about carbohydrate foods. What they are, why runners need them, and how to choose the best ones for you. So, make yourself comfy, grab a cuppa and a slice of toast (yes, bread is predominately carbs!) and read on when you're ready.

What are carbohydrates?

Carbohydrates are one of the three macronutrients, the classes of food your body needs lots of, and they are one of the main ways the body obtains energy for running. Carbohydrates, so called because they contain carbon, hydrogen and oxygen, are an important part of a healthy, balanced diet for runners and non-runners alike. Carbohydrate foods are sugars, starches and fibres that are naturally found in vegetables, grains, fruit and milk products.

When it comes to energy for running and, indeed, all forms of physical activity, carbohydrates are your main fuel source, although not the only one. Carbohydrate fuel comes from the fact that the body breaks down most sugars and starches into glucose, a simple sugar that it can easily use to provide essential energy. Glucose is stored within the muscles and liver as glycogen, so it's readily available for working muscles to use as we run and exercise, by releasing essential energy quickly on demand.

Why female runners need carbohydrates

Female runners need to eat carbohydrate foods for energy. The process of eating it and using the resulting energy works brilliantly when we consume enough to keep our muscles filled with glycogen, but when muscle glycogen stores diminish and are not topped up, the essential energy that all runners need is just not there. You try to keep running but your body says no, which is when tiredness kicks in, you feel sluggish and your running starts to lose its sparkle. Without sufficient energy, the potential for injury also increases.

Because your body gets energy from carbohydrate foods, they are an essential part of a healthy runner's diet. Have you ever tried running for any length of time after a few days of eating very low carbohydrate meals? These may include tasty suppers such as a cheese and ham omelette or a steak and salad, which, though healthy, predominately contain protein and fat, with just a little carbohydrate in the salad. Health wise, you may feel completely satisfied eating like this because they are nutritious meals. However, with a limited carbohydrate intake, it is impossible for glycogen stores to be fully preserved, so as soon as you start running the energy availability from your muscles will be limited. This can lead to early fatigue and underperforming. Following an extremely low carbohydrate diet also has the potential to result in poor recovery, increasing the risk of injury and infection.

What about the flipside of eating a diet consistently high in carbohydrate? That too can leave you feeling sluggish, often from bloating and weight gain, particularly if you over consume nutrient-poor white carbohydrate foods, such as processed white bread and pastries. Carbohydrates are necessary for energy, so eating some is good, but don't overdo it. Once again, as unexciting as it may sound, it is all about finding the right balance.

To get the right amount of carbs into your diet always think about the training session you are doing. If your run is likely to take less than 90 minutes then over-eating carbohydrates beforehand could be detrimental to your performance and possibly result in unwanted weight gain in the long-term. When glycogen stores in the muscles are maximised, the amount of water your body carries increases. It is thought that for every gram of glycogen deposited, an additional 2.7g of water is stored. This means that if you have 400g of glycogen stockpiled, around 1000g – or 1kg – of extra water is also stored in your body. This may not sound like a lot, but you may well feel it during your training.

Types of carbohydrates

The quality of carbohydrate foods varies wildly. For a simple example, think about a sweet potato versus a croissant. Both are sources of carbohydrates, yet one is packed full of vitamins and minerals while the other is high in saturated fat and low in vitamins. One medium sweet potato and one regular croissant each contain almost 30g of carbohydrates, but the nutritional value and the type of available carbohydrates are not equal.

Carbohydrate foods can be referred to as simple or complex. The difference comes from the number of molecules each food is broken down into when eaten and digested. Simple carbohydrates are single or double sugar molecules, called monosaccharides and disaccharides. Glucose is one type of monosaccharide, and fructose and galactose are the other two. Our bodies can easily and quickly digest and process simple carbs, which is why glucose is so readily used for an energy boost.

Fruit and dairy products are also simple and quickly absorbed forms of carbohydrates. One key difference between the varieties of 'simple' carbs is their nutrient value. Fruits are rich sources of vitamins, minerals, fibre and antioxidants, while dairy products offer some protein, vitamin D and calcium. Table sugar and honey offer little, if any, other health benefits.

Complex carbohydrates are made up of longer chains of sugar molecules, and foods like wholegrains, beans and pulses fall into this category. These foods are great for when you need lasting energy rather than a quick burst.

Another way that carbohydrate foods are ranked is by their glycaemic index (GI), which indicates a carbohydrate food's overall effect on blood glucose levels. Slowly absorbed foods have a lower GI rating, while foods that are more quickly absorbed and, therefore, raise blood glucose levels have a higher GI rating. For example, honey has a much higher GI than broccoli. Because whole fruits are digested and absorbed more slowly than fruit juices, due to the fibre they contain, the GI of fruit is much lower than fruit juice and causes less of a rise in blood glucose levels.

More recently, carbohydrate foods have started to be categorised by their nutritional benefits. Terms like 'nutrient dense', 'nutrient poor' and 'high fat' are used to distinguish between carbohydrate food options.

Nutrient profiles of carbohydrates:			
Carbohydrate category	Profile	Foods	Uses
Nutrient-dense	Provides vitamins, minerals, antioxidants and fibre.	Starchy vegetables, beans, pulses and wholegrains.	These foods should form the bulk of your carbohydrate intake.
Nutrient-poor	Provides minimal nutrients.	Energy gels, sugar, sports drinks, white bread and pasta.	These foods should not form a major part of your daily diet but may be useful to provide a compact source of carbohydrate around training sessions.
High-fat carbohydrates	Contain significant quantities of fat, in addition to carbohydrates.	Cakes, crisps, pastries and biscuits.	These foods should be consumed only occasionally and avoided around training sessions.

How many carbohydrates do runners need?

There is no simple answer to this question. Your ideal carbohydrate intake depends on several factors, including training intensity, your daily activity level, your genetics, age, and more.

Gender also plays a role. Men and women require different amounts of carbohydrates. In general, studies show that men use a much higher ratio of carbohydrates for energy than women, while women tend to use more fat. Put simply, to produce a similar intensity run, men need more carbohydrates. Although this is the general pattern, do not forget that we are all unique.

The chart below provides a rough guideline for the daily quantity of carbohydrates that you might benefit from consuming per kg of body weight (/kg BW), depending on your level of activity.

Exercise intensity	Quantity of carbohydrate per day
Light exercise intensity (e.g., walking, yoga, Pilates), once or twice a week.	2-4g /kg BW
Moderate exercise intensity (e.g., running, strength training), up to 1 hour per day.	3-5g /kg BW
High exercise intensity (e.g., endurance running), 1-3 hours per day.	5-7g /kg BW
Very high exercise intensity (e.g., endurance running, triathlon training), 4-5 hours per day.	Up to 8g /kg BW

Here is a practical example so you can see how this could work in real life. A 70kg (11st) woman running three times a week at an easy pace for around 40 minutes a time would require around 3g of carbohydrates per day per kg of body weight.

---

3 x 70kg = 210g of carbohydrate per day.

Thinking in real food terms, here are some examples of how 210g of carbohydrates could be achieved:

- » 2 bananas (50g)
- » ½ can of chickpeas (20g)
- » 100g wholemeal pasta (75g)
- » 50g porridge oats (30g)
- » 100g butternut squash (12g)
- » 100g raw carrot (10g)
- » 200ml full-fat milk (9g)

The foods listed total 206g of carbohydrates.

Of course, you could achieve the same carbohydrate quantity by eating a large bag of Liquorice allsorts (140g of carbohydrate) and 12 Rich Tea biscuits (70g of carbohydrate). Though undoubtedly tasty (I adore liquorice!), these choices would not be useful in providing sustained energy or essential fibre, vitamins and minerals.

What this all means

There are many options for consuming carbohydrates, including vegetables, beans, pulses, rice and oats. As you know, we are unique beings, so I suggest that you choose the type of carbohydrate that not only suits your running training but also suits you. For example, if you are gluten intolerant then eating pasta and bread on a regular basis should be avoided. Ideally, you want to be eating a variety of carbohydrate foods each day, as every food has a slightly different nutrient profile. Variety will give you the best chance of a maximum range of nutrients, which equates to a healthy body and strong running.

> The key point to take away is that yes, carbohydrate foods are essential to running well, and the quantity, type and quality you consume is fundamental to your health and performance.

Protein

The second vital macronutrient you need to know about is protein. Runner or not, this is necessary for everyone, because it is responsible for the growth and repair of every single one of the cells in your body. As a reminder, it is perfectly possible to run well and be in optimum health on either a plant- or meat-based protein diet, or a combination of both. It's up to you to find the most helpful type of protein for your health and performance.

Here you will learn all about protein: what it is, why female runners need it, what happens if you do not eat enough or too much, and how to go about choosing the best protein sources for you.

What is protein?

Protein foods are made up of various combinations of amino acids. When your body digests and breaks down protein foods, these combinations are used to build muscle, bone, tendons and all four types of body tissue. Amino acids also function to produce enzymes that are responsible for transporting nutrients around your body. As such, they are crucial to optimal health, and consuming sufficient protein is vital to both your general health and your specific running performance.

Protein is crucial for the recovery and repair of muscles, as it is a key component of your tendons, ligaments and muscle fibres. During intense exercise, muscle fibres are broken down. Eating protein foods before and after going for a run helps you to counteract this breakdown, and the amino acids in protein encourage muscle repair and growth. Generally, protein foods are consumed after exercise, however, there is emerging evidence for its possible use as a fuel source.

Amino acids

There are 20 different amino acids, each with their own unique function. Some are considered essential, meaning they must come from the food you eat. Others can be produced in the body and so are classed as non-essential, meaning they do not need to come from your diet.

Animal-protein foods, such as eggs, meat, fish and dairy, contain all the essential amino acids and are known as 'complete sources' of them. Plant-protein foods don't contain all the essential amino acids and are, therefore, called incomplete sources. But never fear, there are ways of getting around this. A full range of essential amino acids can be achieved through eating certain combinations of plant-based foods. Examples include brown rice with beans or hummus with wholewheat pitta, both of which are tasty and easy to implement. A well-rounded, plant-based diet will provide adequate amounts of essential amino acids and can provide your body with sufficient protein for effective recovery and repair.

Getting the whole range of amino acids is important for female runners. Although some have more specific benefits than others, they are all needed in their own way.

Why female runners need protein

For female runners, the branched-chain amino acids named leucine, isoleucine and valine can be extra beneficial, because they make up a good proportion of the amino acids located in lean muscle tissue, which gives the all-essential power when running. Within muscle tissue, these branched-chain amino acids work together to help develop and grow high-quality muscle tissue, especially following exercise.

The amino acid lysine is generally only found in small quantities in plant foods, so vegan athletes need to pay particular attention to getting enough through their daily diet. It helps with the production of carnitine, a nutrient that aids the conversion of fatty acids into energy, moderates cholesterol levels and produces the fibrous protein collagen. Therefore, lysine is especially useful for increasing energy levels in female runners. To give you a little bit of perspective, a 60kg (9st4lb) runner requires around 2200mg of lysine per day, based on standard RDA advice. Half a cup of lentils or tofu provide about 600mg each, 1 cup of quinoa or a quarter cup of pumpkin seeds contain around 400mg each. You would have to eat all of the above on any given day to achieve the total RDA of lysine. This is perfectly possible, of course, but it does require some thought and planning.

Sources of protein

This is the fun bit. Getting your taste buds going by talking about all the many different protein sources available. Meat, fish, beans, pulses, nuts, seeds, dairy, eggs and the foods that come from these products, such as tofu, hummus and nut butters are all sources of protein, giving you plenty of choice whatever your taste and ethical preferences. Research studies have found that most moderately active adults who follow a healthy, balanced, non-faddy diet naturally meet protein requirements.

> 20g of protein is a sensible portion size at main meals for most female runners

This could be achieved from any one of the following:

- » 3 large eggs
- » 250g tofu
- » 75g tin of tuna
- » 100g salmon or mackerel

- » 240g can chickpeas or beans
- » 60g chicken or turkey
- » 600ml cow's milk
- » 60g feta or cheddar cheese
- » 60g nuts

Female runners following more plant-based diets need to be aware of the differences in the protein content of cow's milk alternatives. I am not saying that one type of milk is necessarily better than the other, just that there can sometimes be a misconception that they offer the same nutritional benefits.

Plant milks have many and varied health benefits, but decent quantities of protein are not one of them. Awareness around food choice is vital for everyone. The more knowledge you have the more empowered you can be to make the best possible decisions for you and your health and training requirements.

Approximate protein content per cup of milk:	
Cow's milk	8g
Soy milk	6.5g
Cashew milk	4.5g
Oat milk	2g
Almond milk	1.5g
Coconut milk	0.5g

Protein powders

My sporty nutrition clients often ask me about the benefits of protein powders. These are a relative newcomer to the world of sports nutrition and can be a suitable source of protein for some runners, primarily because of their convenience. While I believe in the importance of focusing predominately on real food rather than powders and commercially bought drinks, for certain athletes, protein powders do have their place in a healthy diet.

As the name suggests, they are powdered forms of protein that come from plants (soybeans, peas, rice, potatoes or hemp), eggs or milk (whey or casein). The most biologically available protein in powder form is whey protein, and pea protein for vegans. For anyone on the go with limited access to a kitchen or fridge, protein powders do have a distinct advantage over real food. Post-race, protein powders in shake form really come into their own.

How much protein do female runners need?

As with carbohydrate consumption, protein recommendations are based on quantities per day per kg of body weight. The latest thinking is that protein pulsing, which involves consuming smaller quantities at more regular intervals, is the most beneficial way for athletes to consume protein. Logically, this does make sense and can be easier to fit into a standard day than eating larger portions of protein less regularly.

The current recommendation is to consume 0.25g of protein per kg of body weight 3-6 times a day. For a 60kg (9st4lb) runner, this works out as 0.25g x 60kg = 15g of protein during each meal or snack. That's a third of a chicken breast, a couple of eggs or 4 tablespoons of almond nut butter for each serving.

Over time, not eating enough protein can contribute to loss of muscle mass and strength, a slower metabolism and increased fatigue, none of which is desirable for anyone, let alone a runner with training to do and goals to hit. Although one or two days of consuming lower amounts of protein is unlikely to do any harm to your body, having a low protein intake regularly over a longer period can cause the unwanted effects previously mentioned. Muscle cramps and soreness can increase, which, as well as being painful, may put you off from continued running and possibly leave you more susceptible to illness and injury.

What this all means

Now you know the basics of protein: what it is, why you need it as a female runner and how best to consume it. Protein foods are fundamental to both health and running performance, but unless you have a specific health need or training goal, there's really no need to be too concerned about how much you are getting, as most women consume plenty.

For a greater insight into how and when protein is best consumed for effective recovery after training, head to Section 2.

Fats

Fats are the third and final macronutrient, and they are an essential part of a healthy, balanced diet for female runners. Amongst other things, they are necessary for energy and for transporting vitamins and nutrients around the body.

Before I go into detail about the different types of fats and which ones you should focus on, here's a brief history of our relationship with dietary fat.

History of dietary fat

In the 1950s, researchers found that high levels of dietary fat increased total cholesterol, in turn negatively impacting heart health. This information formed the 1980s guidelines to minimise dietary saturated fat, which is found in butter and full-fat dairy foods. Consumers were steered towards choosing manufactured, low-fat products such as margarine and skimmed milk, bringing about a whole generation of low-fat devotees, who believed that cutting down on fat would be the magic solution to weight loss. But low fat was not and is still not the answer.

Research has hugely evolved and opinions on saturated fats have changed. We now know that for most people, eating small amounts of saturated fats is far healthier than consuming loads of processed 'fake' trans fats, the type found in margarine and other processed products.

More recently, it has been recognised that low-fat foods generally contain higher levels of sugar, which adds to their flavour and makes them more palatable. There is a brilliant if a little heavy-going book called *Salt, Sugar, Fat: How the Food Giants Hooked Us* by Michael Moss, which talks about the 'bliss point' of food and how manufacturers have sucked us in. It's worth a read if you want to get more of a background on the complexities of sugar and fat.

Why female runners need fat

There is no question that dietary fat is a useful energy source, especially during endurance training and events. Research shows that ultra-endurance runners tend to consume more fat than athletes competing in shorter distances. It can be helpful to think about fats as a backup fuel source for when your carbohydrate stores have depleted; fat stores, unlike carbohydrate stores, are almost unlimited in the body.

Lower intensity exercise, such as a long, slow Sunday morning run, relies more heavily on dietary fat than carbohydrate as a source of energy. By increasing the body's reliance on fat as fuel while simultaneously decreasing carbohydrate reliance, in theory, fatigue can be delayed and endurance performance increased. Does that work in practice? Yes. Several studies have shown that time to exhaustion is significantly improved when endurance athletes consume a medium-to-high-fat diet as opposed to a low-fat one.

When you begin to run at a faster pace, your body relies less on dietary fats to keep you going, instead switching to carbohydrate use. Research indicates that female runners are less able to maintain high intensity running on a higher fat, lower carbohydrate diet. However, do not take that as meaning that if you only run shorter, faster distances you can get away with ditching fat from your diet completely and simply eating all the carbs in sight. Dietary fat is vital for healthy skin and for hormonal and brain function. Always consider your overall health as much as your running goals.

As with everything to do with nutrition, the ideal percentage of daily dietary fat and the perfect balance between unsaturated and saturated fat is unique to each one of us. This is because female runners vary in terms of how much fat they metabolise. All female runners need to eat some carbohydrates and some fats, but the ideal ratio for you is individual, depending, amongst other things, on your training goals and genetics. Experimentation, testing and an element of intuition as to what suits you best for the training you are doing and the life stage you are at is needed.

Some runners don't consume sufficient healthy types of fat. That was me back in my 20s, when my diet was primarily based around white carbs, sugar and alcohol. Although there is no one-size-fits-all magic quantity of fat to eat, it is known that low-fat diets over long periods of time can result in vitamin deficiencies and low energy, leaving you susceptible to illness and injury. Before the age of 30, I certainly suffered with erratic energy levels and persistent running injuries.

All female runners need some fat in their diet because it is necessary for balanced hormone function in addition to energy production. Chapter 3 goes into greater detail about female hormones and the vital role that diet plays.

Fat-soluble vitamins

There are four fat-soluble vitamins, so called because they dissolve in fats and oils rather than in water, as other vitamins do. These are vitamins A, D, E and K. Fat-soluble vitamins are necessary for runners because they help bone metabolism, immune function and tissue repair.

Fat-soluble vitamins, their functions and food sources:		
Vitamin A	Vitamin A plays a key role in maintaining your vision as well as supporting immunity, maintaining fertility and encouraging cell and hair growth.	Vitamin A is mainly found in foods from animal sources, but it can also be derived from carotenoids, such as beta carotene, which is found in red and orange-coloured vegetables. Effective conversion, however, is dependent on genetics.
Vitamin D	Vitamin D is the sunshine vitamin, so called because it is produced by your skin when it is exposed to sunlight. Like vitamin A, vitamin D supports healthy immune function, but is also well-known for its beneficial effects on bone health. This is because it regulates circulating calcium and phosphorus.	There are two major forms of vitamin D: D2 and D3. Mushrooms are a great source of D2, while D3 is found in eggs, fish oil and sunlight.
Vitamin E	Vitamin E is a powerful antioxidant, protecting cells from premature ageing and damage from free radicals. These antioxidant properties are enhanced by other nutrients, such as vitamin C, vitamin B3 and selenium. In high amounts, vitamin E also acts as a blood thinner, reducing the blood's ability to clot.	Vitamin E is found in sunflower seeds, almonds, wheatgerm oil and green leafy vegetables.

Fat-soluble vitamins, their functions and food sources:		
Vitamin K	Vitamin K plays a key role in blood clotting. It also supports bone health and can be beneficial for the heart.	Leafy green vegetables and soy products are great sources of vitamin K.

Dietary fat helps the body to absorb these essential, fat-soluble vitamins. Something as simple as drizzling a colourful salad with a little olive oil can help increase your absorption of vitamins. You should think of fat as your vitamin friend.

Types of dietary fat

As with carbohydrates, not all fat is created equal. For women, the type of fat regularly consumed is especially important.

Broadly speaking, there are four kinds of fat:

» Essential
» Good for us
» Bad for us individually
» Downright unhealthy

Essential fats are also known as essential fatty acids (EFAs). Strictly speaking, there are only two true EFAs, namely linoleic acid (LA) and alpha-linoleic acid (ALA). LA and its derivatives are omega-6 fatty acids, while ALA and its derivatives are omega-3 fatty acids. Getting the right balance of omega-3 and -6 is crucial, as omega-6 tends to be more pro inflammatory, meaning these fats can promote inflammation in the body, while omega-3 essential fats are anti-inflammatory, helping to reduce unnecessary inflammation. We need both types of essential fats, and finding the balance between the two can be tricky. Generally, it is much easier to consume omega-6 essential fats, while omega-3 fats require a little more thought to obtain.

Omega-6:	Omega-3:
» Sunflower oils » Soya beans » Meat, eggs and poultry » Processed foods	» Oily fish, such as herring, sardines, salmon and mackerel. » Nuts and seeds, such as walnuts, chia seeds and flaxseed.

The second type of dietary fats are those that are good for us. These are plant-based fats, such as avocado, avocado oil, coconut and coconut oil, as well as organic, grass-fed meat and dairy products. These types of fat have many health properties, which are good for your heart, brain, skin and, crucially for runners, for providing essential energy.

Thirdly, there are those fats that are bad for us individually. Remember the fact that we are unique – there is no magic ideal diet that suits everyone. For example, nuts and seeds provide a daily source of essential fats for many women, but those of you with nut allergies have to avoid them, and for some they can even be fatal. As another example, some people find it difficult to tolerate fat in red meat, while others have no problem with it. When selecting food sources for your daily dietary fat, always keep in mind your wonderful individuality.

The final type of dietary fat are those fatty foods that are downright unhealthy. Here, I am talking about trans fats, also called trans-fatty acids, which is a type of unsaturated fat that is used in the manufacturing of processed foods to increase shelf life and stabilise flavours. Consuming too great a quantity of trans fats can raise your 'bad' cholesterol, which is associated with an increased risk of heart disease. This type of fat is predominately found in packaged cakes, biscuits, snacks and fast food. My advice is to avoid these foods whenever possible; they will not help you run faster or stronger, and neither do they offer any health benefits.

Not all fats are 'bad'. It used to be thought that fat was the enemy, but we now know different. However, this message still needs to get across to some women, who have spent most of their adult lives limiting their fat intake. Our diet as a whole is contributing to increased obesity rates throughout the Western world, it is not solely the quantity of fat we consume that is to blame. However, that does not mean we can tuck into as much cream and butter as we like. Eating too much fat, especially of the less healthful type, is no doubt detrimental to both our wellbeing and our athletic performance.

How much fat do female runners need?

As already explained, women need a good supply of the fat-soluble vitamins A, D, E and K, and the fat we eat helps us to absorb these essential vitamins.

UK health guidelines recommend that the average woman aged 19 to 64 should eat no more than 20g of saturated fat per day. Women who take regular exercise, including running, are not immune to these basic health recommendations, so do not be fooled into thinking that because you train on a regular basis you can get away with eating more saturated fat. The odd meal or day of eating higher fat does no real harm, but on a regular basis it is best to stick to the guidelines. Too much saturated fat contributes to higher levels of cholesterol and weight gain, both of which are likely to impact your running performance.

Based on a moderate fat Mediterranean-style diet, you could be eating upwards of 60g of fat per day, mainly monounsaturated fat from olive oil, nuts and seeds.

One medium-sized avocado contains around 30g of fat. So too does 60ml of double cream. The difference is the type of fat in each of these foods. Avocado is about 20g monounsaturated fat, a heart-healthy fat, and 5g each of polyunsaturated and saturated fat. Double cream, on the other hand, is mainly saturated fat. It only takes about 40ml of double cream for you to hit the recommended maximum daily intake of saturated fat. You would have to eat a whopping four avocados to hit this peak.

Fat content in typical foods, highlighting the difference between processed and unprocessed foods:	
One skinless salmon fillet	8g of fat
One tbsp of ground flaxseed	3g of fat
10g of butter (enough to thickly cover two slices of bread)	8g of fat
Regular bar of dairy milk chocolate	14g of fat
200ml of whole milk	7g of fat
One Gregg's sausage roll	22g of fat

What this all means

Healthy types of dietary fats, such as olive oil, avocados, nuts, seeds and oily fish are essential for female runners. You need them for your muscles, skin, hormones and a strong performance.

Do not scrimp on the gorgeous healthy fats available for fear of gaining weight. That is an old diet myth that needs dispelling.

Sugar, alcohol, hydration

The sweet stuff

Mmmm . . . sugar! Who doesn't like a hit of the sweet stuff every now and then? A couple of sugary biscuits, a piece (or bar) of chocolate or a scoop of ice cream from your favourite local shop (hands up, that is one of my favourites, especially after a summer run along the river!). These sugar kicks can turn your day from bleh to great in the blink of an eye. And as for those yummy gummy sweets handed out during running races, how can they not fail to put a smile on your face when your legs are hurting, and you are wondering why on earth you ever decided to sign up for this crazy race in the first place?

In this part of the book, you will learn about sugar in all its forms. This includes the benefits and the downsides, because as with a lot of foods, there is no simple wrong or right. I'll explain the different types of sugars found in foods, which ones are the most useful for runners, and which can negatively impact both your health and your performance.

Once eaten, all forms of sugar move from the stomach into the liver, where they are transported into the bloodstream before moving into the cells of the body. In an ideal world, this process happens at an appropriate rate to meet energy needs and keep your blood glucose levels stable. When glucose hits the blood, it stimulates the pancreas to release insulin, which then triggers the uptake of the glucose by the body's cells (e.g., muscle cells), causing blood glucose to return to base levels. Insulin release turns off fat burning, instead promoting glucose burning as the body's primary fuel source. Finally, any excess glucose ends up being stored as glycogen in the muscles. When storage capacity is reached, any extra glucose is stored as fat in your fatty tissue.

The benefits of sugar for female runners

There is no denying that glucose, the substance that carbohydrate is broken down into, is an important fuel source for your body. In basic terms, because sugar is absorbed so quickly, it gives a well-needed instant boost of energy that can be vital immediately before or during a run. Other types of food, such as meat and high-fat meals and snacks, take much longer to be absorbed into the blood stream and become available for your body to use.

Research indicates that the effects of the sugar eaten before or during a run may be more pronounced in female runners than in male ones. The reasons for this are currently unclear, but studies show that female hormones play a role. For women, elevated blood glucose, which happens after eating sugar, disrupts hormone production. This can negatively impact many areas of your health, such as your fertility, menstrual cycle, weight and mental wellbeing.

These problems undoubtedly have a knock-on effect on your running performance. Chapter 3 explains in greater depth the impact female hormones have on running performance and nutrition choices.

The downsides of sugar for female runners

Several studies have reported increased levels of GI distress, in the form of diarrhoea, stomach cramps and nausea, in women who consume refined sugars immediately before and during exercise. GI distress is also reported to occur more frequently and more severely in those runners who consume energy gels containing refined sugars during races and training (remember that sugar doesn't just come from food, it is also found in sports drinks, energy gels and other sports nutrition products). Fructose, which is the type of sugar found in fruit, irritates the stomachs of some runners. If this is the case for you then try to avoid eating fruit and foods containing fructose in the few hours before running and during training.

Another downside of consuming too much sugar is the resulting cravings. These tend to indicate reactive hypoglycaemia – low blood glucose – in the same way that feeling irritable or having poor concentration if a meal is missed does. You will know if that is you. It is that grouchy, short-tempered feeling we all hate. Sugar cravings are no fun, as they make you feel like the only way to get going again is to have another hit of sugar. Of course, eating some sugar can do the trick temporarily but the downside is that it can leave you feeling worse than before and looking for your next 'hit'. Eating refined sugars too often or in large quantities in one go causes large highs and lows in blood glucose levels, which has the potential to trigger further sugar cravings. It can become a rollercoaster of ups and downs, leaving you dependant on sugary foods and eating too much for optimum health.

Different types of sugars

There are many different forms of sugar. So many, in fact, that it can feel like a confusing minefield. Here, I'll share with you everything you need to know about different forms of sugar, plus their corresponding benefits and downsides to you as a runner.

Let me start with fake sugar. Artificial sugars are the chemical substances, usually calorie-free or low-calorie, that are found in chewing gum, toothpaste, fizzy drinks and processed foods like cakes and desserts. Artificial sugars that have been approved for use in the UK, at the time of writing, include aspartame, saccharin, sorbitol, stevia and xylitol. The question is: does your body react to these chemicals differently to how it would to sugar? Certainly, there is a difference in terms of taste, and research suggests that the excessive consumption of artificial sweeteners may stimulate appetite and play a role in weight gain and obesity. However, the research is inconsistent and, therefore, the links between artificial sugars and obesity are somewhat inconclusive. It does seem that artificial sugars do not increase blood sugar levels to the same extent as natural sugars, which may be of benefit to some runners. With both pros and cons to artificial sugars, you need to find out what works best for you.

Natural sweeteners, such as coconut sugar, maple syrup, honey and molasses can make great substitutes for refined cane sugar. The most important point to make here is that just because they are more natural foods and less refined does not necessarily mean they are healthy for you. Consuming all forms of sugar in moderation is vital, as it is just as possible to gain weight and suffer from health issues as a result of eating an excess of honey as it is caster sugar.

Natural sweeteners generally have additional health benefits that refined sugar lacks. For example, molasses is rich in iron, honey has antibacterial properties and coconut sugar is packed full of potassium and magnesium. However, as far as your body is concerned, they are still sugar.

Sugar can be shown on an ingredients list as any of the following:

Corn syrup, dextrin, dextrose, high-fructose corn syrup, honey, lactose, malt syrup, maltodextrin, maltose, rice syrup, saccharose and treacle.

Energy gels

A staple for many longer distance runners, energy gels can provide an essential boost and stave off fatigue during longer runs.

There are different types of gels available, so do try them out to discover which ones suit you best. Also see my review of them on page 150.

Traditionally, energy gels are made with simple refined sugars, however, sports nutrition is a booming market and in recent years a variety of more natural ones have become available. You can now find honey-based gels, chia seed gels containing coconut sugar and a touch of pink Himalayan salt, and even gels made from dates, maple syrup and brown rice syrup.

I know many runners, myself included, who no longer want to consume traditional energy gels. Equally, there are some female runners who aren't concerned with the type of sugar they eat during a run, as their thoughts are purely focused on the energy it provides. Whatever your own thoughts on the matter, why not try making your own energy gel? It's not as difficult as you might think.

Here's a simple recipe you could try:

How to make 150ml of energy gel:

» 1 tbsp chia seeds, ground
» 60ml water
» 4 fresh Medjool dates, stones removed
» 3 tbsp fresh lemon juice
» 1 tsp pink Himalayan salt
» 1 tsp blackstrap molasses

Method:

In a small bowl, gently stir the ground chia seeds into the water and set aside for around five minutes to allow a thick gel to form.

Meanwhile, combine all of the remaining ingredients in a food processor or high-speed blender until everything is mixed together.

Once the chia seeds gel has thickened sufficiently, add it to a food processor or blender and mix until a smooth, gel-like consistency has been obtained.

The gel can be stored in a container and used during your next long training run.

How to reduce sugar in your daily diet

"Eat less sugar, you're sweet enough already." - Unknown

Reducing sugar for health reasons mainly involves steering clear of added sugars where possible. As already mentioned, fruit, dairy and other carbohydrate foods are naturally broken down into sugar molecules in the body. These are natural and most people do not need to cut them out of their diet completely. Refined sugars, which are the ones found in cakes, biscuits, chocolate, processed foods and the sugar you add to your cup of tea or coffee, are the ones you would benefit from minimising.

But how? One of the simplest ways of reducing refined sugars is by swapping white starchy carbs for their wholegrain alternatives. That means replacing white pasta with wholemeal pasta and switching white bread, bagels, pittas, wraps, etc., with their wholemeal counterparts.

Secondly, you could avoid or cut right back on cakes, biscuits, sweets, chocolate and other processed goodies. This is easier said than done, perhaps, but if you are serious about improving your health and running performance it is most definitely doable. Think about making different choices. For example, if you and your family like a sweet treat, try home baking with brown rice syrup, honey or dates. These are still forms of sugar, so moderation is key, but they do have some goodness in them. Remember to base your meals around protein foods that are satisfying and keep you feeling full.

For various health reasons, some of you may need to avoid sugar more than others, but all of us could do with monitoring our intake and making healthier choices when we're not training. Sugar can be of benefit during long training runs or races but consuming it in excess may result in health problems and reduced performance.

What this all means

Natural forms of sugar, in moderation, can be your friend when running and exercising intensely. You can use sugar to your advantage by fuelling long runs and replenishing muscle glycogen immediately afterwards. Outside of training, though, it is better for your overall health to avoid artificial sugars and refined white carbohydrate foods as much as possible.

Alcohol

I find that views around the subject of drinking tend to divide female runners. Some women I have spoken to feel that drinking alcohol on a regular or sporadic basis has no impact on their health and running performance. They are more than happy to have a few G&Ts or glasses of wine the night before a race or a long run. Other women know for sure that alcohol is not good for their health or their running and avoid it as much as possible. Perhaps you fall firmly into one of these camps, or maybe you have managed to strike a happy medium.

Certainly, as I have gotten older, I see and feel the impact that drinking a glass of wine or two has on my sleep, mental function and energy levels the next day. I am currently at that point where I can still drink but want to less and less.

In this section of the book, I'll share the latest research around alcohol consumption in relation to female health and athletic performance, giving you the essential facts and empowering you to make your own informed decisions.

Variances on the effect of alcohol

It is well known that there are large variations in the effects that alcohol has on individuals. Factors such as genetics, gender, the amount of alcohol drunk at any one time, body mass and nutrition status go some way to explain these variances.

Your body mass and the size of your liver are two factors in how much alcohol you can break down and eliminate in an hour. However, recent research has shown that your genetics could be one of the most significant factors in how you deal with a tipple or two. People with certain genetic variants tend to be slower metabolisers of alcohol, which means they are more likely to experience its negative side effects, such as distorted vision and speech. This is because the alcohol stays in their body for longer.

Impact of alcohol on health

In terms of health, there is no doubt that alcohol can be detrimental, which is partly due to the fact it is so calorific. A glass of prosecco contains around 120 calories, while half a bottle of wine comes in at around 350. Because there is no nutritional value to alcohol, it is simply empty calories. Additionally, alcohol calories are not converted to glycogen like carbohydrate foods are, so they provide no fuelling benefit and are not an appropriate source of energy for your body during exercise.

Rather than being converted into glycogen, the body turns energy from alcohol into fatty acids, which is stored in your fat tissue. Essentially, this conversion process means that alcohol consumption increases fat storage, impacting your percentage of body fat, which obviously isn't useful for your running performance or health. Although alcohol is undoubtedly an enjoyable relaxant for many of us, it has no major health benefits for runners, whatever your gender.

A recent study suggested that middle-aged men can see a positive result from consuming moderate quantities of red wine, as it results in increased levels of 'good' HDL cholesterol. However, the same study found there was less of a benefit for middle-aged women.

Impact of alcohol on performance

Most runners sensibly abstain from alcohol the night before a race, but a celebratory drink afterwards seems to be a different matter. Many of us love a cold beer or two after completing such a challenge, especially on a hot day. I have two vivid memories of drinking alcohol after a race. The first was a very cold beer on Brighton beach after finishing a tough and extremely hot marathon in 2011. That beer was utter bliss and was accompanied by the best fish and chips ever! My other alcohol-after-racing memory is of a pint of local ale while lying in a field with a bunch of other sweaty, knackered runners after my second 60km ultramarathon. That was one fine, well-earned beer!

Alcohol as a means of celebration or relaxation after a special run is fine on occasion. However, if you are in the middle of a serious training plan, rather than toasting the completion of a race think more carefully, because research indicates that drinking alcohol after exercise means you are less likely to follow optimal post-run nutrition guidelines. Plans tend to go out of the window after drinking, something I am sure you have experienced at one time or another. Drinking too much alcohol after a run prolongs your recovery, so you may not be sufficiently rested and repaired before your next training session or race. If immediate alcohol intake is inevitable, I suggest you strive to only consume small volumes and always match one boozy drink with a glass of water to counteract the dehydrating effects.

Obviously, drinking too much alcohol results in a hangover, which is never pleasant. This will undoubtedly impact the next day's training session, though studies show that some athletes frequently consume alcoholic drinks without much consideration for the chronic long-term effects on performance and health.

Alcohol is a diuretic, meaning it increases fluid loss from the body by encouraging the kidneys to produce more urine. Extra fluid loss can lead to dehydration, one of the symptoms of a hangover, which ultimately delays recovery. Excessive alcohol is toxic to the body, requiring massive amounts of processing by the liver. Research indicates that aerobic performance capacity decreases by up to 11 per cent when hangover symptoms such as nausea, low mood, headaches and soreness occur.

Research shows that another reason why drinking alcohol impacts recovery, both mental and physical, is that it can negatively affect sleep patterns. A glass or two of wine may help you fall asleep faster and possibly sleep more deeply for a short time, but it will significantly reduce overall restorative sleep – REM sleep – which is so vital after intense exercise. Read on to Chapter 10 for much more on sleep.

Alcohol and nutrition

Research shows that chronic, excessive alcohol consumption leads to nutritional deficiencies in all women regardless of activity status, specifically of the B vitamins, including B12, folate and thiamine. These vitamins are needed to metabolise carbohydrates into energy, in addition to the formation and maintenance of healthy red blood cells vital for endurance running. This means that regularly drinking alcohol can leave you feeling low in energy and in no way ready for a decent running session.

Finally, studies have shown that long-term alcohol use diminishes protein synthesis, which is the way our bodies use protein to create muscle mass, resulting in a decrease in muscle growth. Even short-term alcohol consumption has the potential to negatively impact your muscles, due to its dehydrating effect.

What this all means

Alcohol is not going to improve either your health or your running performance. However, away from training and competition, it can certainly be enjoyed by most in moderation and as part of a healthy, balanced diet.

You are now armed with the essential facts and it is up to you to make your own informed decisions.

Hydration

Starting each run sufficiently hydrated is hugely important for all runners, male and female alike. Remember, though, we aren't simply 'small men', so we need to approach hydration in a different way to them, instead of simply drinking a bit less.

It is thought that there are differences in the balance of sodium and fluid in men and women, which is mainly due to the menstrual cycle and associated oestrogen and progesterone hormones. Women have less body fluid than men, which means you can feel thirsty many miles before your male counterparts during the same race conditions. But don't necessarily take this as a sign that you should be drinking more plain water while running. Here, I'll explain why, and exactly what you do need to include in your hydration plan.

What is hydration?

Hydration is the process of replacing water in your body, which can be done through drinking water and other fluids or by eating foods with a high water content, such as cucumber, tomatoes, celery and apples. Dehydration occurs when more water is lost than replaced. Over time, this leads to your body not having enough water to be able to function properly.

A completely accurate picture of your hydration status is difficult to determine out of a lab setting. But there is one very simple test you can do yourself and in the comfort of your own home. Next time you use the toilet, simply have a look and check the colour of your urine. Ideally, you are looking for a pale, straw colour. Darker colours indicate some degree of dehydration. You will find a link to a urine colour chart in the resources section at the back of the book.

Please note that if you take vitamin supplements that include riboflavin – vitamin B2 – then bright yellow urine is a common side effect, so do not be alarmed. Beetroot can give your urine a pink tint, while asparagus is famous for producing distinctive-smelling urine in some people.

How dehydration affects health and performance

Dehydration happens when your body doesn't have as much water as it needs. Long term, this makes you feel rotten and unable to function properly. The most common symptoms are feeling thirsty, a dry mouth, headaches, lethargy, dizziness and dark-coloured urine.

Dehydration primarily impacts your health; your running performance is secondary. Research reveals that running speed and perceived exertion (how fast you think you are running) are impacted by even mild dehydration. Basically, not taking on enough fluid slows you down and makes each step you take feel harder than necessary.

Even low levels of dehydration can have physiological consequences. A loss of 2 per cent bodyweight, which is 1.5kg for a runner weighing 70kg (11st), increases perceived effort and may reduce performance by between 10 and 20 per cent. That is significant. Fluid loss exceeding 3 to 5 per cent bodyweight considerably reduces your aerobic exercise performance by worsening reaction time, judgement, decision making and concentration.

Hydration for runners

Is it OK for female runners to just drink plain old water before and after running? This is fine if you are only going for a few miles at an easy pace and the weather is not too hot. But for some runners, staying hydrated can be a little more complicated than simply drinking tap water. Do you ever get a salty taste on your skin or lips after exercising, especially in hot weather? Well, that is sodium loss. The sweat your body produces contains salts and minerals, as well as water, therefore, it is important to replenish your body with salts as well as water.

Electrolytes

Salts and minerals excreted in sweat are called electrolytes, which are located in your blood. The main electrolytes are sodium, chloride, potassium, magnesium and calcium.

Sodium

Sodium is the main salt in your sweat. It plays an important role in regulating the total amount of water in your body, and it is critical for functioning well. Too much sodium raises your blood pressure by holding onto excess fluid in the body, creating an extra burden on your heart, which increases your risk of a stroke or heart failure. On the other hand, too little sodium in your body, known as hyponatremia, is equally dangerous.

Hyponatremia in runners results from having surplus fluid in your body relative to a normal amount of sodium. It usually occurs after drinking an excess amount of plain water while not replacing the electrolyte salts you've sweated out. Symptoms of hyponatremia include weakness, headaches, nausea and muscle cramps, making you feel shaky and disorientated.

Research indicates that women are much more vulnerable to the risks of hyponatremia than men while endurance running. The reason for this is partly because a woman's body doesn't contain as much water, even when their BMI is the same as a man's. This means it takes less water intake to dilute extra cellular fluid in the body. Slower runners are more at risk of hyponatremia than those at the front of the pack. This is simply because they have more time and opportunities to drink water excessively.

Potassium

Potassium works to help regulate fluid balance, muscle contractions and nerve signals, as well as being helpful for lowering blood pressure. Low levels of potassium in your diet have the potential to cause weak, cramping muscles.

Good sources of potassium include bananas – a favourite of many runners – spinach, other leafy greens and potatoes.

Calcium and magnesium

Calcium and magnesium work together for powerful muscle function as well as strong bones. Muscle cramps, spasms and twitches are common effects of low calcium and magnesium, in addition to sore muscles and, for some women, trouble sleeping.

Nuts, seeds, wholegrains, leafy greens and dark chocolate all contain good quantities of magnesium. For calcium, dairy products are the obvious choice, but almonds and sesame seeds, bony fish and cruciferous veg (broccoli, cabbage, sprouts) are also helpful sources of calcium.

Hydration during running

The whole running nutrition business has boomed in recent years, meaning there are several options on the market to help boost your hydration during runs.

Salt tablets that you chew or leave to dissolve in your mouth are convenient and easy to carry around. They only contain essential electrolytes, so there's no carbs or sugars. When taking these types of tablets, it's important to sip some water to help get them absorbed properly into your body.

Some hydration tablets need dissolving in water before drinking. These are great for convenience and come in a variety of palatable flavours. Some contain extra ingredients, such as caffeine and vitamin D, which aid calcium absorption. Try some different ones out to discover the ones that work best for you.

Finally, the other essential, practical thing to get sorted for staying hydrated during runs involves how to carry your water. For shorter distances when you are starting your running journey, handheld water bottles can be fine, but over longer distances you ideally want to be running handsfree. This is when hydration vests and packs come into their own. They are a great way of carrying essential fluids, as well as food and other bits and bobs needed during a long run. Just resist the temptation to pack too much in – you have got to carry it all as you run!

Hydration after running

Drinking plain old water will replace lost fluids, but as already explained, it will not help you with replenishing lost salts. One simple solution is to add a quarter of a teaspoon of quality Himalayan salt to a large glass of water, which quickly and efficiently replaces lost salts. Another option, especially useful on a cold day, is to stir a teaspoon of Marmite, Vegemite or Bovril into hot water to make a delicious salty drink packed full of B vitamins, which are vital for energy production. A hot Marmite drink is my absolute favourite thing after a winter run.

Coconut water, the clear liquid found inside a coconut, is naturally rich in sodium, potassium, calcium, magnesium and phosphorus. In a dream world, we could go for an early morning run on the beach, collect a fallen coconut and crack it open right there in the sunshine. In real life, though, the only practical option (unless, of course, you do live on a desert island) is to buy coconut water from the shops. The main thing to consider is what else has been added to the drink, so I recommend checking the label and choosing a brand with no added sugar in any form. There are some out there, it is just a matter of spending a little time looking.

If you like to eat fluids as well as drinking them, a watermelon can be a great choice, as it also contains good levels of electrolyte minerals. On some of the ultramarathons I have done in hot weather, slices of watermelon and other fruits were available at the feed stations – they were a welcome sight.

Milk is another popular and useful drink to enjoy after running. I know there is a lot of controversy around the health benefits and risks of regular cow's milk, but from a hydration point of view it does the job well. This is partly because cow's milk also contains a suitable balance of carbohydrates and protein, which, as I have already explained, are essential for your recovery.

What this all means

What and how much you drink is just as important as what you eat. In some situations, this is even more so the case. The combination of water and electrolytes is invaluable for female runners, whatever the weather and distance you run, so make sure you prioritise fluids as much as food.

CHAPTER 3

HORMONES

"A healthy outside starts from the inside." - Robert Urich

Hormones are chemical messengers that act like an internal communication system in your body. They play a role in many of your bodily activities, including your metabolism, appetite and fertility. The 'dance of your hormones' is a delicate one. The two main protagonists I will focus on in this chapter are the female sex hormones oestrogen and progesterone. I will discuss their role in the monthly menstrual cycle, PMS and the menopause. There are a whole host of other hormones at play in your body, some of which I touch upon in other chapters, but oestrogen and progesterone are the two most relevant and researched for female runners.

There are many associations with female hormones and the impact they have on exercise enjoyment and performance. It is beyond the scope of this book to go into every condition individually. Your monthly cycle, which I'll talk about next, is a good place to begin because it forms the basis of everything else. You will come to see that some foods, such as sugar, are mentioned time and again in terms of how imbalanced they can make your mood and energy, while other foods, such as leafy greens and EFAs have the opposite effect in many situations. These foods form the basis of a healthy, happy hormonal diet.

When sharing knowledge about any subject, it always helps if you can hold your hand up and say, "I've been there, I know how it feels," And I can. Monthly cycle hormonal fluctuations and PMS haunted me for many years. These were the years I struggled with menstrual cramps, bleeding on inconvenient days, breast tenderness and mood swings. Casting my mind back to these less-than-pleasant times is not nice, but I do take comfort from knowing that everything I went through was normal for a woman of my age at that time. Thankfully, in some ways, I am now heading away from these monthly cycle and PMS trials and into a different stage of life, the perimenopause. Now, I am not sure if this is going to be less challenging or more, as women transition through this time of life in different ways. I will just have to wait and see. As with all chapters of this book, nutritional information with regards to female hormones is based around the latest scientific research. Let's get you running through your current stage of life feeling awesome and strong.

Menstrual cycle

On average, women spend about 40 years of their life going through the menstrual cycle, and up to 10 years of that can be spent on your period. These numbers highlight exactly how important talking about the monthly menstrual cycle is. It forms a significant part of your life, so dealing with it in the healthiest way is a significant step forward.

The menstrual cycle may affect different aspects of your running performance at different times of your life. For example, severe abdominal cramps and heavy blood flow can interfere with engagement in exercise, while, at the other end of the scale, excessive exercise and dietary restriction can lead to recurrent injuries and a complete absence of your period. I want to ensure that women like you are able to run, exercise and perform at your absolute best whichever life stage or phase of your monthly cycle you are in.

What is the menstrual cycle?

The menstrual cycle is the time from the first day of a woman's period to the day before her next one. The average is a 28-day cycle, but longer or shorter ones – anything between 21 and 35 days – are completely normal. Cycle length can also significantly vary month on month. If this is the case for you then rest assured that it can be normal and healthy. However, irregular periods can be a sign of starting the perimenopause or a medical condition such as PCOS or low thyroid function. If you have any concerns, please do contact your GP for a check-up to see what the cause might be.

The menstrual cycle is a hormonal dance involving oestrogen, progesterone, follicle-stimulating hormone (FSH) and luteinising hormone (LH). The first half of the menstrual cycle (days 1 to 14 in a 28-day cycle) is termed the follicular phase, and this is when levels of oestrogen rise, causing the ovaries to produce follicules. Ovulation, when the growing follicle is ruptured and an egg is released, occurs on around day 14 of a 28-day cycle, in response to a surge in LH.

The second phase is termed the luteal phase. It usually occurs between days 14 to 28 of a cycle, and at this point the hormone progesterone increases, helping the womb to prepare for the implantation of a developing embryo. If pregnancy does not occur, the egg is reabsorbed into the body, levels of oestrogen and progesterone fall, and the womb lining comes away and leaves the body as a period, signalling day 1 of your next menstrual cycle.

How the menstrual cycle affects running performance

Performance during the monthly cycle varies widely across female runners, and age and other factors such as stress levels also play a role.

Hormonal fluctuations can affect how you process the food you eat, your energy levels, sleep quality and the severity of your sugar cravings. Plus, there can be uncomfortable physical side-effects, such as bloating and changes in breast size, to contend with. Any of these changes can make consistent training more challenging.

Research studies conducted in Europe during the 1960s painted a depressing picture. They found that more than half of the female participants experienced a reduction in exercise performance during menstruation, specifically when it came to how long they could exercise before exhaustion and how intense the exercise was. However, on a more positive note, recent studies found no differences in a woman's ability to exercise at any point in the menstrual cycle. Note, though, that there appear to be some exceptions to this, as longer distance running events – marathon distance upwards – resulted in slower times for women who ran during menstruation. Whatever formal research studies find, bear in mind that they are usually done in a controlled setting. In real life, many women, including myself, do experience changes in how running feels, whatever the distance, at different times of the month.

Cyclical training

Often, the first few days of menstruation can be a more challenging time to run. Training cyclically, by planning harder and longer training sessions around your menstrual cycle, may be the answer. This way of training can be especially useful for recreational runners who aren't tied to high-level competition dates. It is certainly something that I have done in the past. I used to take a few days off running the day or two before my period was due, making sure I had done my longer or tougher training on other days of the month. The best way to plan cyclical training is to look at your typical menstrual cycle and schedule in longer, harder training sessions on the days when your energy levels tend to be higher, which could be from around day 5 to day 23. Energy levels generally peak around the time of ovulation, so you may find that running can feel brilliant at this time. Make the most of it, because it could be an excellent time to go for a personal best. Factor in less intense training sessions from around day 24 to day 4 of your next cycle, because these tend to be the days where energy levels are lower and pre-menstrual symptoms occur. You will know your body best and I urge you to listen to it. Remember that we are all different so don't be afraid to experiment and see what works best for you.

Try not to panic if a race you have entered and have been training hard for falls on an inconvenient day of your monthly cycle. A positive mindset is key to success. Call it mind over matter if you like. Any increase in stress and anxiety will negatively impact your mind as well as your body. Thinking yourself into a positive place where you will be able to run well is a great start. The nutrition aspect is also important, of course, and is covered next. As I mentioned earlier, some studies reported slower marathon times for women who were racing during their period. However, other studies disagree. They found no evidence to show that there are variations in muscle glycogen concentrations throughout the menstrual cycle. Obviously, you need to take into account the practical side of things when running for several hours during your period, but with some thoughtful planning this should not be an issue.

Body temperature

Another way your monthly cycle can affect your running is through changes in body temperature. It is well known that a woman's core body temperature varies according to the stage of the menstrual cycle she is in. Women have a higher core temperature in the second half (luteal phase) of the menstrual cycle due to the thermogenic heat-producing effect of the hormone progesterone. This increased body temperature makes your breathing and heart rate increase, which for runners produces extra stress on an already stressed body.

This happened to me when I ran my second ultramarathon during an unexpectedly hot April day. By the time my friend and I had reached the last checkpoint, with just 5 miles left to go, after 7 solid hours of running, my core temperature was way too high. My heart rate rocketed and remained extremely high despite the fact we were only moving at an easy jogging pace. It took plenty of walking breaks plus taking on a lot more salt and cool water to get my heart rate down to a manageable level, but I must admit it was a scary experience. The race was a few days before my period was due and I do think that played a role in how my body responded to the heat on the day. If you find that core body temperature increases during the second half of your menstrual cycle impact how you cope with runs on hot days, ensure that you incorporate electrolytes and hydration into your diet.

Fuelling during the menstrual cycle

Finally, let me explain how hormonal levels during your menstrual cycle influence the types of fuel your body uses for energy.

During the first half of your cycle – the follicular phase – more oestrogen is produced. Because of this, your body more readily conserves glycogen stores and has an increased ability to burn fat. Strength training also has more of an effect, so it is a great time to lift weights. During intense training and races, you do need to be extra careful to take in enough carbohydrate, around 40g per hour. Regular protein is also necessary, plus an increase in iron-rich foods like red meat, apricots, leafy green vegetables and beans help to replace recent blood loss.

The second half of your cycle – the luteal phase – produces an increase in progesterone. At this stage, your metabolic rate increases along with energy expenditure. Your body also switches to being more fat-dominant, so this could be a good time to slightly increase your consumption of healthy fats such as nuts, avocados, olive oil and oily fish.

Common menstrual cycle issues and how to support them through nutrition

Heavy periods

Heavy periods are a common, distressing problem for many women, and they are one of the most common reasons for seeking advice from a medical practitioner. They can feel debilitating and make exercising uncomfortable and stressful. They also impact energy levels and can result in iron-deficiency anaemia, which is associated with slower running speeds and reduced endurance capacity. What you eat can help manage the symptoms from heavy periods. Good nutrition includes iron-rich foods such as apricots (dried and fresh), spinach and other leafy greens, lentils, beans, red meat and egg yolks. As blood is so rich in iron, the loss of it results in lower levels being available for your body to use, and these foods will help to replenish your levels and increase vital energy for running.

Menstrual cramps

My own menstrual cramps always felt like a constant, painful throb, making me feel irritable and uncomfortable. I used to struggle to find the right foods and drinks to soothe my stomach and not irritate it further. Foods that have been well studied in relation to relieving menstrual cramps include bananas, walnuts, ginger, fish, leafy green vegetables and pineapple. You may benefit from basing your diet around these foods on the days you are on your period, as there is enough evidence to say that it could make a significant difference. Ginger tea is something I highly recommend. It is an effective, soothing drink that could ease cramps without interfering with your running performance. You can either grate a little ginger into hot water, with a squeeze of lemon, or go for the convenience of tea bags. One reason why pineapple can be effective for menstrual cramps is that it is high in the mineral manganese. However, be mindful, as some women report that eating large quantities can bring on their period earlier. This is thought to be due to one of pineapple's active ingredients, bromelain, which is a known muscle relaxant. Undoubtedly, pineapple has antioxidant properties that can calm acute inflammation and ease cramps. There are also practical things you can do to relieve your discomfort, such as using a hot water bottle or giving yourself a gentle tummy massage.

Amenorrhea

At the other end of the scale to heavy periods and cramps is amenorrhoea, a complete absence of the menstrual cycle. This can result from a combination of excessive exercise and dietary restriction, and it's more common than you might think in female athletes. In order to return to a healthy menstrual cycle, your body needs sufficient nourishment and calories, especially from healthy fats, calcium-rich foods, vitamin D-rich foods and protein. Additionally, because your mindset and mental health can be an underlying reason for the temporary cessation of your periods, I suggest you also read

Chapter 5, which focuses on good mental health in female runners.

Oral contraceptives

How do oral contraceptives affect running performance? Some can cause weight gain and bloating, making training feel more of a struggle than it used to. However, we all have individual reactions to contraceptives and there are many alternative birth control options.

Currently, there is not much research on the effects of hormonal birth control on running speed and endurance, partly because of the difficulties in gathering accurate data. Of the research that has been published, some suggest that birth control use may have a small, negative impact on strength gains, Vo2 max and aerobic capacity in elite athletes. However, other studies have not backed up these claims and so the evidence remains inconclusive.

It is not all bad news for hormonal contraceptives. They have been shown to lessen cramps and reduce heavy periods for some women, which can improve their enjoyment of running and may increase speed and distance as a result.

Discussion around the menstrual cycle and exercise is important. I believe that the beauty and joy of women like you is your ability to conceive, to care for others, to feel strong emotions, to have the mental strength to train and smash your goals and to empathise with other female runners. That is your power. Your fluctuating female hormones make you the amazing woman you are.

PMS

Following on nicely from the topic of the female menstrual cycle comes PMS. It is a rare woman who has never suffered with at least one symptom of it at one time or another.

Premenstrual Syndrome (PMS for short) is the name for a collection of symptoms that can occur in the days before menstruation begins. It is linked to changes in hormone levels, and research suggests at least 85 per cent of women experience symptoms to some degree every month. However, women may not share the same symptoms or have them to the same degree every single time they menstruate. I have always suffered with premenstrual breast tenderness and spots, but the emotional symptoms have varied widely. For instance, my diet has a huge impact on my mood. On those rare occasions I eat junk food, my mood drops, and I feel more anxious and out of control. On the other hand, when my diet is based around whole, healthy foods, I feel calmer and happier.

Emotional PMS symptoms:

- » Depression
- » Mood swings
- » Anxiety
- » Irritability
- » Tearfulness
- » Changes to sex drive and appetite

Physical PMS symptoms:

- » Bloating
- » Headaches
- » Breast tenderness
- » Spots
- » Greasy skin and hair

How PMS affects running performance

From a practical viewpoint, physical PMS symptoms, such as bloating and tender breasts, can make running extremely uncomfortable, with the added challenge of clothing. I know more than one runner who has different running kits for various points in their menstrual cycle. They tell me that leggings with looser waists and bigger running bras can be a godsend.

Emotional PMS symptoms have the potential to be improved by running and exercising, which is great if you can motivate yourself to get out of the door. Many women understand the benefits of going out for a run but find that getting started is their biggest challenge. Feeling tired and low during the lead up to your period can make even the most disciplined woman struggle to keep up a regular routine. This is where goals, accountability and support come into their own. When you have a clear goal, such as an event to train for, people to check in with you, sponsorship money to raise or someone to run with, you stand a much better chance of overcoming emotional PMS symptoms and getting out there.

How diet and PMS interact

I have already mentioned how my own diet has the potential to play havoc with how my symptoms manifest. Associations between diet and PMS are complex, and there isn't one single type of food or way of eating that either causes or can stop all your symptoms. The impact of what you eat is unique and individual to you. However, there are some foods that have been proven to increase the symptoms of PMS, and others that, in general, help women to sail through relatively unscathed.

Because PMS is linked to changes in hormone levels, balancing hormones through diet and lifestyle is paramount.

Sugar

The top food linked to PMS symptoms is sugar. Consuming an excess causes elevated levels of glucose and insulin in the blood. In turn, this disrupts hormones, which leads to physical and emotional symptoms in the weeks before your period. If you notice that the amount of sugar you eat impacts your PMS symptoms then make a conscious effort to reduce your intake of foods containing refined sugars, such as white bread and concentrated fruit juices.

Chocolate cravings are commonly associated with PMS, and they are linked to low levels of magnesium. Essentially, we crave what our bodies need. Regular milk chocolate is packed full of refined sugars and contains little magnesium. Dark chocolate is the way to go to satisfy premenstrual chocolate cravings because it contains good levels of magnesium, antioxidants and phytonutrients. A bar that contains 75 per cent cocoa is good, or, if you like a strong, bitter taste, go for 90 per cent.

Stimulants

Adrenal stimulants, including caffeine, alcohol and nicotine, play havoc with female hormone function. Adrenal stress is a major factor in PMS and other hormone-related issues, so by cutting out or reducing these stimulants you will be placing less stress on your adrenal glands. Although the occasional glass of wine or coffee may not do too much harm to your health or running performance, regularly relying on them isn't good for your stress levels and hormones.

I do appreciate that it can be easier said than done to cut out these addictive stimulants. I adore my daily coffee, but sometimes it doesn't adore me. I find that by having a smaller amount of the good stuff, be that coffee or wine, my body and mind become more resilient and PMS symptoms fade.

Foods that support PMS

Some foods have been shown to reduce the severity of PMS symptoms.

Firstly, high-quality protein, such as poultry, eggs, fish, lean meat and beans and pulses, can be useful in supporting you through this time, partly because they are rich in vitamins B1, B2 and B6, which have been shown to reduce PMS symptoms by up to 35 per cent.

Foods containing friendly bacteria are also your PMS friend. Kefir, yoghurt, sauerkraut and kombucha are readily available options that you might want to try. For the best results, aim to incorporate a portion of these foods and drinks into your diet daily during the second half of your monthly cycle. Prebiotic foods, such as asparagus, leeks, onions and garlic, help to feed the 'good' bacteria in your gut, so try to include them too. One word of caution is to start incorporating these foods into your diet slowly, because if you are unused to eating them they can cause temporary bloating and gas.

Magnesium, known as nature's relaxant, is one of the most vital nutrients for managing PMS symptoms. Magnesium-rich foods include pumpkin seeds, squash, spinach, Swiss chard, fish such as halibut, and nuts and seeds. Several studies have shown that an increased magnesium intake can effectively reduce bloating, headaches and breast tenderness. Additionally, magnesium is also proven to aid a good night's sleep, which in itself can help with managing and reducing PMS symptoms.

Hydration is another important element to PMS, as drinking plenty of water is a vital and often overlooked element for healthy hormone function. Water helps with hormone detoxification, plus it is necessary to transport all the wonderful nutrients in your food around your body. Whether or not you are planning to go running, it is important to remember to drink water throughout the day.

So, there you have it. What PMS is, why it can stop you from running and some of the things you can put in or take out of your diet to help. If you suffer with PMS, you may not necessarily need a complete dietary overhaul; it may be that some small tweaks make enough of a difference. I suggest you start by choosing one or two things to try and keep a record of how successful the changes are.

Menopause

There comes a time for most women when PMS symptoms start to fade. *Excellent news!* you may be thinking. And yes, it is great when you don't have to deal with periods and monthly cycle fluctuations anymore. However, the reason why periods and PMS dwindle is because the menopause is kicking in, which can bring its own challenges. Menopause, which literally means the pausing of menstruation, is the term most widely used, but in fact there are two distinct parts: the perimenopause and the menopause.

Perimenopause is the lead up to the menopause. It is a transitional phase beginning several years before the change occurs. Your ovaries will begin to produce less of the hormone oestrogen, causing changes that cascade through your body. The perimenopause typically starts when a woman is in her 40s, but it can be earlier, and just as with PMS, women experience it differently; some sail through it, others suffer immensely.

Menopause occurs when your ovaries produce so little oestrogen that you stop ovulating and your periods cease. The average age for a woman to reach the menopause in the UK is 51, but remember this is the average – you may hit yours some years either side. In less developed countries, the menopausal age tends to be lower, due to different lifestyles and diets.

Running through the menopause

Women who already run and want to continue doing so throughout their perimenopausal years may have an advantage over those of you who started later in life. Women who have been running and exercising for longer by this stage have great base health and fitness levels that will stand them in good stead to thrive during these transitional years. But if that's you, don't get too complacent. Hormonal fluctuations can hit any of you, whatever type of runner you are. Believe me, I know.

Women who take up running and other forms of exercise later in life can most definitely reap huge benefits. It is never too late to improve your health. Whatever age and fitness level you are at right now, just get started. You won't regret it.

Just like with PMS, there are a collection of symptoms related to the perimenopause and menopause. You may suffer with some worse than others, while some may bypass you completely. There is no telling how the menopause will affect you.

Hot flushes

Hot flushes are one of the most common symptoms women experience during the perimenopause, and for runners they can be a real problem. This isn't just down to the fact you can experience one right in the middle of an already sweaty run, but also because of the intense tiredness that often accompanies them.

Hot flushes affect your running performance in several ways, the main ones being fatigue and dehydration. Changes in hormone levels affect your body's temperature control and your internal thermostat stops working properly. Hot flushes feel like a sudden heat spreading through your body, usually accompanied by a red flush moving across your chest and face, an increased heart rate and sweating. This all feels particularly unpleasant and uncomfortable during a run.

Nutrition for hot flushes

There are a few nutritional strategies that have research backing up their use for moderate hot flushes, which I'll talk about in this section.

When blood glucose levels naturally drop between meals, some women find hot flushes appear quicker and more intensely. If this happens to you, make sure you eat regular meals and consume healthy snacks, as they'll keep your blood glucose levels balanced and lessen the likelihood of the hot flushes occurring. The best way to balance blood glucose levels is by prioritising lower GI carbohydrates, such as whole grain rice and pasta, beans, lentils, chickpeas, green vegetables and lower-sugar fruits. These foods minimise blood glucose spikes and dips that could trigger hot flushes.

Watch out for post-run dips, also called reactive hypoglycaemia, as it is common for blood glucose levels to drop for several hours after intense or long-duration exercise. This is due to your body becoming more sensitive to insulin. The action of exercise draws on glucose stored in your muscles and liver, called glycogen, and while your body goes through the process of restoring it, glucose is taken from your blood. Low blood glucose levels are possible even up to eight hours after a long or strenuous run, and the more intense your activity, the longer your blood glucose will be affected. Studies show that consuming a low GI meal or snack before running can reduce the release of glucose, minimise low blood glucose levels and produce smaller fluctuations over the course of a day. This simple action could make all the difference when it comes to menopausal hot flushes. Additionally, your post-run snack is just as important as what you eat beforehand. Things like a piece of fruit or a granola bar are great for gently returning blood glucose levels to a more normal amount.

Finally, consider your intake of the following minerals, which play a vital role in how body cells interact with insulin.

Nutrient	Food sources
Chromium	Broccoli, brewer's yeast, seafood, wholegrains, brazil nuts and pears.
Zinc	Red meat, chicken, nuts and seeds.
Copper	Shellfish, dark chocolate, mushrooms and sweet potato.
Magnesium	Leafy green vegetables, almonds and dark chocolate.

When you consume a sufficient supply of these minerals, the pancreas releases insulin in a more measured way and your body becomes more effective at absorbing and using sugar. This moderates highs and lows in blood glucose and may help to reduce hot flushes.

Caffeine

There are other triggers for hot flushes in menopausal women. Caffeine, the active component of coffee and tea, is known to cause a rise in body temperature in some women. If you find this happens to you then herbal teas, of which there are many, can be a wonderful alternative to caffeinated coffee and teas. Sage tea has been frequently researched and proven to help many women with controlling hot flushes. It is well worth trying out different herbal teas and keeping a stash of your favourites handy in the kitchen.

Phytoestrogens

There is good evidence that phytoestrogens, which are plant-based oestrogens that mimic the effect of our body's own oestrogens, can help reduce the severity and frequency of hot flushes. Isoflavones, a well-studied type of phytoestrogen found in soy, legumes, lentils and chickpeas, have been found to reduce the intensity of hot flushes. But how can you make the science work for you in practice? Aim to eat one portion of beans or pulses every day. If daily feels a touch too far then try alternate days. If you tend to follow a vegan diet then beans and pulses may be a staple food already, but if these are new to you then go slow. Take it one meal at a time because your body, especially your gut, may take time to adjust to these new foods.

Omega-3 essential fatty acids

Only 7 per cent of Japanese menopausal women report hot flushes, compared with up to 80 per cent of women in the UK. On average, Japanese women consume 1,300mg of omega-3 fatty acids per day, while in the UK, the average daily intake is only around 200mg. The numbers say it all. Omega-3 is vital for hormone function, through making them, transporting them around your body and balancing out levels, and research suggests its properties help with reducing the frequency and intensity of hot flushes.

Omega-3 fatty acids include EPA and DHA, which are found in oily fish, and ALA from plant-based foods like flaxseeds and chia seeds. ALA can be converted into beneficial DHA within your body, but this conversion process is not necessarily efficient and can be poor in many women. This is where genetic testing can help, by pinpointing exactly how your body processes and converts the foods you eat.

Current UK government guidance is for women to consume 1,100mg of omega-3 fatty acids every day.

Sources of 1,100mg omega-3:

» One portion of oily fish (sardines, mackerel, salmon, herring and anchovies).

» One tbsp of flaxseed or chia seeds, or their oils

» Eight walnut halves

If you do not get enough omega-3 through the food you eat, consider taking a supplement. There are many options, whether you prefer fish oils or seaweed-based vegan supplements. If in doubt, get in touch with a registered nutrition professional such as myself to talk through the best options for you.

Dietary symptom triggers

The food and drink triggers of perimenopausal symptoms can be vast and varied, mainly because we all experience this stage of life differently. However, there are some commonplace triggers that appear to affect many women.

Spicy foods, alcohol, caffeine, sugar, stress and smoking can all trigger hot flushes. It is a very personal story, though. An Indian takeaway may have you stripping off a layer or two and glugging down gallons of water, while your friend may be fine with a vindaloo. Personally, I am slowly coming to the sad realisation that red wine can trigger a hot flush. Even just one small glass leaves me red-faced and sweaty.

What this all means

One way to keep an eye on the extent to which what you eat and drink might be impacting hot flushes and other symptoms is by keeping a food and drink diary and recording the side-effects you experience alongside it. This can really help to pinpoint the triggers.

Of course, sometimes symptoms will occur for no obvious reason at all, but if you can find a pattern then great. Always remember that you are unique and, therefore, have your own distinct set of circumstances that trigger menopausal symptoms.

In summary, no matter how horrible hot flushes and other menopausal symptoms make you feel, remember the benefits of running. Research backs up the thinking that aerobic exercise tends to reduce the severity of symptoms. So, in light of this awesome news, keep on running!

CHAPTER 4

RUNNING TO LOSE WEIGHT

Many women start running with the goal of losing weight rather than getting fitter. There is a long-held belief that intense exercise, of which running is one option, leads to weight loss. For some women, this can be true to a certain extent, but to see the most gains in health, fitness and weight management, running does need to be combined with dietary changes.

> The interactions between running and weight loss are complex and include genetics, the people you choose to spend time with, and, perhaps surprisingly, restricted eating.

Genetics

Here, Dr Eve Pearce, Scientific Officer at myDNAhealth, the award-winning nutritional genomics and epigenetics company, discusses the role of genetics in relation to running and weight loss. Founded in 2014, myDNAhealth uses advanced DNA testing combined with lifestyle analysis to offer in-depth reports, giving the vital information needed to make positive lifestyle changes that are perfectly adapted to you.

These additions by Dr Pearce have been kindly contributed exclusively for this book.

A brief introduction in genetics

As a species, humans have long looked to predict their future, with questions such as: "Is our health predetermined?" or "Can we change our fate?" Following the discovery of DNA (famously identified by James Watson and Francis Crick in 1953), some thought that our destiny might be written within it. The DNA double-helix concept is now well-recognised and consists of two DNA strands wound around each other, a bit like a twisted ladder. The DNA strand itself comprises alternating combinations of four 'building-block' nucleotides, split into 23 different divisions, known as chromosomes. Spread across these are instructions (known as genes) for the proteins that make up our tissues. Each individual inherits a combination of genes from both their parents, which account for the diversity we can see across the human population, and the similar traits that can run in families.

The Human Genome Project (HGP) was a ground-breaking international scientific research collaboration. Researchers across the globe worked towards a united goal of determining our entire DNA code. The project got underway in 1990, with the high aspiration to fully understand our genetic code and how it has influenced us. By 2003, the project was complete, giving us the first map of our chromosomes. It revealed that the human genome has just over 3 billion nucleotides, making up the DNA code of our 23 chromosomes. It was a historic achievement!

One of the big surprises to come out of the HGP was that we have far fewer genes than was originally estimated. In 1990, it was thought that due to our complex biology and vast numbers of expressed proteins, we were likely to have up to 100,000 genes. However, less than a quarter of human genes have been identified. To put this into perspective, bread wheat contains over 105,000 genes compared to roughly 25,000 human genes. The project was conceived to answer the mysteries of our genetics definitively, but instead, learning our DNA code has opened up more questions. Scientific research has since moved onto investigating how our genes are expressed into different proteins, which function together to make up our cells and tissues. So, whilst our unique genetic code alone isn't the fortune teller we had hoped for, we do know that it has a considerable influence on our health.

The shift towards personalised nutrition intervention for health and wellness

Since the completion of the HGP, our understanding of the complex interactions between our diet and lifestyle and our genes has progressed considerably, using genetic data. Precision Nutrition (PN) is a relatively new way to use the information we continue to find out about our genetics. It works by combining knowledge from the two main aspects that make us who we are: our unique DNA code and our environment. Utilising both can work to fully optimise diet and lifestyle advice and promote health, wellness and fitness. This personalised understanding can also improve the motivation to change behaviour, which can be a crucial barrier to lifestyle or dietary intervention.

What does Precision Nutrition genetic testing involve?

The human genome is predominantly the same in all of us, with less than 1 per cent of our DNA code being different. The majority of these small differences involve just one nucleotide change in our DNA sequence, known as SNPs (pronounced 'snips'), which account for many of our genetic traits. Most commercially available genetic tests analyse DNA to look for SNPs that are related to health. At myDNAhealth, we embrace the philosophy of PN, using both well-researched genetic SNPs and questionnaire information to personalise nutritional and lifestyle advice. The Optimal Health report analyses a selection of carefully chosen genetic traits, which make up the slight variations in our DNA.

This information combines with in-depth lifestyle questionnaire data to present individualised nutrition and lifestyle advice in a user-friendly online platform.

The genetics of running and weight management

There are a variety of reasons why people choose to take up running, and one of these might be for weight management. If we use a simple calorie in-and-out model, to lose 1lb of fat, you have to burn approximately 3,500 calories. Depending on your size and running speed, this could take a few hours. But, whilst this is a popular goal, running does not always equal weight loss. Why is this? One of the questions that researchers have been exploring is: "Do our genetics hold the answers to why running is more effective for weight loss in some than others?" Well, the answers are complex, and it's not just about your workout routine or one single genetic variant. As part of the optimal health product, we recognise that body weight is influenced by a range of factors, such as appetite and eating behaviours related to energy balance and metabolism.

Much of our knowledge about appetite control is derived from studying the genetics of obesity and the altered signalling pathways involved. These can be investigated together to understand the regulation of appetite and body weight. The brain has been identified as the primary appetite controller. It receives and assimilates various signals from the body, such as our external (e.g., exercise) and internal (e.g., fat tissue percentage) environments. Working to determine our overall appetite response (either hunger or satiety), our brains regulate how much food we consume. As energy availability is integral to our survival, it's not surprising that we have powerful hunger signals. The myDNAhealth approach to investigate appetite regulation uses an integrated nutritional genomics-based system. Positively correlated SNPs, including FTO and MC4r, are analysed in combination with detailed lifestyle questionnaires.

FTO

In 2007, two scientific research groups independently identified the first established obesity vulnerability gene. Catchily named the FTO gene (fat mass and obesity-associated gene), it is thought to have the most significant genetic influence on our BMI and, therefore, our risk of obesity. Its role is believed to be in the control of food intake and preferences for energy-rich foods. Those who have a genetic variant in this gene are more likely to be overweight and will be, on average, 3kg heavier. FTO is useful in understanding our genetic response to exercise when it comes to weight loss. Although predisposed to be heavier, those who possess this genetic variation can significantly improve their body weight from aerobic activity, including running. Research has also shown that those who understand their FTO genetic profile and comprehend the benefit of making alterations to their lifestyle instigate more positive changes than those who don't. As they say, forewarned is forearmed.

MC4r

Another gene with a critical role in the satiety response is MC4r, which codes for an appetite-suppressing protein mainly expressed in the brain. MC4r is linked to a wide variety of biological roles, such as weight, cardiovascular function and mood. As it is expressed in the regions of the brain that regulate stress, it is suggested that the combination of MC4r genetic variations and stress influence eating behaviour, resulting in weight gain. Those who have a genetic variant show decreased responsiveness to the appetite-suppressing MC4r hormone, crave fatty foods and store more visceral fat. These tendencies can be reduced by dietary coaching and addressing stress through lifestyle changes such as running, which helps to manage stress hormones

Other factors

As Dr Eve Pearce so eloquently explained, genetic variances play a significant role in health and weight management, being one important piece of the puzzle.

Other factors that can also play a role in weight loss include the people you choose to spend time with and the myth that simply eating less and running more will make you lose weight.

Interestingly, one study undertaken more than 30 years ago showed that friends can have an even greater effect on a person's risk of obesity than our genes. The research found that if a friend becomes overweight, your risk of following suit increases by a whopping 171 per cent. I'm not saying you should start blaming your friends if you find weight hard to shift, however, the social circles you spend time in are worth bearing in mind.

We know that cohabiting partners have an increased chance of gaining weight, which is attributed to feeling secure, loved and happy. Women seem to draw the short straw, being most likely to gain significant weight within a year of moving in with their partner. For men, it appears to take a little longer before this negative effect takes place.

There is a common misconception that low-calorie diets coupled with increased running and other forms of intense exercise make you lose weight. Science simply does not back up this thinking. Time and time again, studies have shown that the combination of consistent reduced portion sizes, resistance training and aerobic exercise produce the best weight-loss results. Consistency is important, as is approaching weight loss with a healthy mindset, meaning that you should be prepared to make realistic changes to your way of eating and exercising that are sustainable and practical. When you cut down on carbohydrates or frequently skip meals in an effort to lose weight, you are not giving your body what it needs to build the necessary muscle. In order to maintain energy levels, glycogen stores must be replenished after every training run, otherwise there is an increased risk of injury or not even making it out of the door for your next scheduled run.

I encourage all runners to run for its myriad benefits, including improved sleep and increased energy, other than solely for weight loss. Reducing stress through obtaining more time outdoors, having meaningful connections with friends and getting in enough hours of refreshing sleep can also contribute to weight loss.

Finally, remember your uniqueness. Don't compare your weight loss, running speed or distance with anyone else's. Do what is best for you and let others be themselves.

CHAPTER 5

MENTAL HEALTH

"Good food warms the heart and feeds the soul" - *A.D. Posey*

Mental health, nutrition and running are inextricably linked. Your mental health affects your food choices, body image, motivation, resilience, and vice versa. Being a healthy person is not just about physical health, as in whether you can run, jump and move comfortably for a prolonged period. Health also incorporates the state of your mind and how positive and motivated, or otherwise, you feel.

The term mental health has been more commonly used since the late 2010s, and it refers to the state, or health, of your mind. It's how you think, feel and behave and it's the words you use and the messages you tell yourself.

What you eat and drink either helps or hinders your mental health.

In this chapter, I'll cover three of the most important areas of mental health for female runners:

1. Mental load
2. Emotional eating
3. Orthorexia

Whatever your situation, please know that you are not alone. We all have times when we feel down, stressed or anxious. Although these feelings often simply pass, sometimes they develop into something more serious, weighing you down for longer. If you feel that this is the case for you, please do seek advice from your GP or another qualified medical practitioner.

> Undoubtedly, what you eat affects your mental health and wellbeing and, consequently, your running performance.

Mental load

Mental load is everything you do, all the tasks you oversee and the responsibilities you take on in order to manage your life. It is also all of the things you need to think about. I use the word 'need' loosely, as potentially some of your mental load can be let go of.

As an example, I like to track and analyse my running. How far, fast, my VO2max, heart rate, elevation and the like. But I don't 'need' to keep on top of my running statistics. When work and family life become busier, I ditch my fitness tracker and simply run for enjoyment. For me, this is one way to reduce my mental load back down to a more manageable level. I know that by tracking my running I am adding to my stress and things to think about.

Thankfully, mental health in athletes is receiving more attention than ever before, as it is in the general population. It is common knowledge that when you are juggling a lot of things, having a greater mental load can impact your health through increased levels of stress, but how does mental load impact running performance in women?

How mental load impacts running performance

Research shows that physical performance is reduced when you are under greater stress. The same goes for decision making and skill execution. It could be argued that running requires much less skill than many other sports. I mean, you just put one foot in front of the other (albeit hundreds of times over!). But decision making when running is crucial, especially when trail running. You need to have your wits about you to avoid tree roots, rabbit holes, deep mud and other obstacles.

Research also shows that the greater your mental load the higher your rated perception of effort, meaning how hard you feel you are working. So, when you've got a lot on your plate, running tends to feel tougher. Although your watch might say your pace is the same as usual, it could feel like you are working harder. When your mental load is high, there can definitely be less of a natural ease to running.

Practically speaking, having too many things to do and think about impacts the time you have available to get out for a run. For example, you might be a mum of two school-aged children, with a part-time job, a husband, a family, a house and pets. That is a lot of responsibility, and there is a good chance that in this type of situation exercise, self-care and time to yourself isn't always going to be top of your priority list. Trust me, though, it doesn't have to be this way. By taking good care of yourself through the right diet and exercise, your mental health can stay in relatively good shape.

If you, like me at times, find that having too much going on means that running and exercise takes a reluctant back seat then see what can be dropped. There is usually something that can be cut short, shifted slightly or even dropped altogether to give you the time and headspace to fit in a run.

Here are my top three strategies to free up time:

1. On a Sunday evening, I will sit down and decide on a plan of lunches and dinners based on what the week has in store. So, I might decide to cook a batch of eggy muffins on Monday lunchtime and store some in the fridge for the following day.

2. Bolognese always goes down well with my daughter, so I might cook that one evening, eating half that day and keeping half for later in the week, with the addition of kidney beans to add some additional oomph.

3. One-tray, oven-baked dishes are my ultimate dinner favourites, including foods like baked fish, sweet potato, roasted peppers and aubergine. By choosing foods that can cook slowly in the oven, I have the time to get a strength training workout or a short hill training session in,

To see what is impacting your own mental load, you could create a life wheel, which is a visual representation of different areas of your life, rated on your level of satisfaction. You can then easily see which areas need working on and which may be taking up more headspace than you would like.

There are two fundamental things related to mental load and running that I realised once I became a mum. Firstly, that you need to put yourself first sometimes, because your needs are just as important as those of your children and the other people in your life. In some ways they are more important.

There is that old classic saying about putting on your own gas mask before helping others. Certainly, I am a nicer and calmer mum if I have exercised and taken some time for myself. And my daughter will vouch for me being less than patient when I've not made the time for even just a short walk around the block or a handful of squats and lunges before dinner.

Secondly, I eventually came to the realisation that it is not possible to give all your time to all the areas of your life at any one point. Think back to your life wheel. Is every single area really a 10/10? If you are ploughing energy into training for a race and a cool work project or two, I bet your social life is less than full. You can't always have it all. Life tends to ebb and flow, so be OK with that.

Stress hormones

There are some key hormones that are well known for being vital players in your stress response. Cortisol is one of them. This is released by the adrenal glands in response to stressors, of which intense running is one, as part of the fight-or-flight reflex. The hormone plays a vital physiological role, providing your body with the energy needed to fight, whether that be to ward off an attack from a wild animal, jump out of the way of an oncoming car or deal with your argumentative child.

Cortisol is also produced in response to injury, illness or infection. Because cortisol has potent anti-inflammatory effects, it does help with easing pain and irritation, however, long-term, high cortisol is not good for your health.

Frequent bursts of cortisol can cause anxiety, poor sleep, irritability, morning exhaustion, sugar cravings and abdominal weight gain. Any one of these symptoms can undoubtedly impact your health, as well as how well you run.

The effects of constant high cortisol are far-reaching. There comes a point when your adrenal glands get worn out and your endocrine system, the collection of glands that produce hormones, is triggered to start finding other sources of cortisol to keep up with demand. In the extreme, your body may 'steal' the steroid hormone pregnenolone, which would ordinarily go into producing other hormones like oestrogen and DHEA (dehydroepiandrosterone, a hormone produced by your body's adrenal glands). In turn, this can impact fertility and growth, so high cortisol can be an issue for female runners also hoping to start a family. The dance of the hormones is real.

There is no doubt that frequent intense running is a severe physiological stressor, indicated by an increase in cortisol production. Racing, a club track session or pushing yourself to the limit during training are all forms of intense exercise, but when you balance out intense running with relaxed miles and calming activities like yoga, stress hormones naturally lower.

What this all means

Mental load boils down to the amount of stress and the things you have going on in your life that result in less time, energy and brain power for running. Sometimes, that does not matter so much, but if you have an event in the diary that is important to you or a fitness goal that is paramount to your health then perhaps something else in your life may need to go. You need to decide what is best for you.

Emotional eating

Emotional eating is a response to stress, unhappiness, pleasure and boredom, and it can be something we use to reward ourselves. It is eating for comfort rather than for satisfying hunger, and for some women it can be a way of coping and shifting thoughts and feelings elsewhere. At times, we all use food to cope with stress, fatigue, anxiety and other uncomfortable feelings. You could say that emotional eating is like giving yourself a big hug with food.

Usually, we emotionally eat with high-fat, high-sugar foods, such as cake, ice cream, biscuits and chocolate. Drinks wise, a nice cup of tea or a glass of wine are common favourites, depending on the time of day.

Perhaps you calm down after finally getting the kids to bed by self-soothing with a large glass of wine. Or maybe you treat yourself to a bar of chocolate after making a difficult phone call or encourage yourself to finish a piece of work with the promise of another coffee and a slice of cake. These are all forms of emotional eating. Indulged in occasionally, this is unlikely to be a problem for your health or running performance, but over time, consistent emotional eating can undeniably be detrimental to both.

At one extreme, emotional eating can trigger an eating disorder. Binge eating disorder (BED) and bulimia have strong associations with emotional eating. If you are concerned in any way, please see the end of this book for some useful resources.

Eating to deal with uncomfortable or unwanted feelings is also strongly associated with weight problems. A person might gradually gain pounds that they then need to shift, or find it difficult to lose unwanted bulk. This can obviously be a problem for both running and body image, as well as your health markers.

My story with emotional eating

Emotional eating and weight gain can be especially problematic when you are injured and on strict, no-running orders, which is something I have first-hand experience with.

In 2020, I went through six months of enforced rest from running while I waited for and then recovered from foot surgery to correct a bunion and two hammertoes. My orthopaedic surgeon was clear that it would take several months for my foot to heal enough for me to do any intense, weight-bearing exercise. After finding even walking painful in the months before the surgery, that was a tough pill to swallow.

Logically, I knew that not running was the right thing to do, but the lack of physical activity took its toll on my mental health and emotional eating kicked in big time.

Because of my nutrition knowledge and training, I did prioritise eating good, healing foods, but there was also much cheering myself up with sweet treats and wine. This was fine in the short-term, but the longer it went on the more difficult the habit became to break. Happily, once I could run again, the emotional eating stopped and I was able to get right back on my usual diet, while fully focused on health and healing.

Factors influencing eating behaviours

What, how much and when we eat are all our free choices to make, which sounds great in theory. But emotions, both positive and negative, can influence our eating behaviours and sometimes override what our head and stomach tell us is a sensible meal choice. When I watch TV in the evening, I often snack on savoury foods. This isn't because I am hungry, it is purely through boredom. And when I am having a stressful day, sugary treats suddenly become more appealing for a feel-good fix.

Certain research indicates that unhappy emotions, such as anger, stress and sadness tend to result in people choosing more sweet foods. But other studies have found that these negative emotions make people crave stodgy comfort foods such as pizza. These conflicting pieces of research show just how personal food choices are. During a stressful day, you may want to devour a block of cheese and a loaf of bread, or maybe you'd prefer a large bar of chocolate. Either way, food choices are driven by emotions as well as hunger and nutritional requirements.

Your running can also impact your food choices. If you hit your training pace, find a gorgeous new trail route or get a new race PB the elated 'high' feelings can lead to celebratory food choices. But if your pace is off, you struggle through your long weekend training run, or don't get the PB you worked hard for, your food choices could be different, veering more towards the comforting and soothing end. Emotional eating comes from positive as well as negative emotions.

Problems with emotional eating

Emotional eating is not necessarily a problem for female runners if it happens only occasionally. For those of you just starting out on your running journey and looking to improve your health and maybe lose some excess pounds, emotional eating has the potential to negate the health and weight management benefits of your new hobby. If you reward yourself with 'treat' food every time you achieve a new running milestone, you could end up gaining weight. It is far better to run for enjoyment rather than reward.

Ultimately, emotional eating doesn't make you feel good about yourself. And this can lead to having a poor body image, which may have a knock-on effect by not making you feel good about your running. Emotional eating is trying to fix uncomfortable feelings with food rather than by dealing with the root cause of what is going on. If you are too busy at work and feel stressed, then getting a takeaway on the way home might give you some temporary comfort, but it will do nothing for resetting tight deadlines and reducing your stress levels a little. And once that takeaway is eaten there is very little chance of you heading out for a stress-relieving run.

Exercise in any form is well known to help with reducing stress levels and improving coping mechanisms for whatever life throws at you. At the same time, using food as a reward aside, it has the potential to reduce comfort eating.

How to curb emotional eating

Firstly, try to become aware of what you are doing and think about what has prompted you to start thinking about food. Has there been a trigger, such as a smell, memory or habit? Perhaps something or someone has upset you or made you feel angry. In which case, it might be necessary to take a few deep breaths to give you some space between how you feel and how you react.

Secondly, use that pause between feeling and action to consider what would feel good in your stomach right now. Imagine how you might feel while eating a particular snack or treat and how it might make you feel later.

What this all means

I'll finish this section with a reminder to ditch the guilt and judgement over your food choices. When you do choose a 'treat', enjoy every single mouthful. Self-acceptance is so important. Aim for a basic healthy diet 90 per cent of the time. This should be based around complex carbohydrates, healthy fats, fresh fruits and vegetables, quality protein and sufficient water, because feeding yourself these fabulous foods will show your body that you are worth it. And you'll also be setting yourself up for strong, healthy running.

Nutrition is one element of treating yourself kindly, with all the love and respect you deserve. There are other ways too, such as meditation, social connection, talking therapies, music and movement, which can help you work through stress and uncomfortable emotions. In

Chapter 11, Clare Flaxen, a CBT (Cognitive Behavioural Therapy) Therapist, explains how to make lasting positive changes to your diet, providing mindset and CBT strategies for eating well and running strong.

Orthorexia

Orthorexia, an obsession with eating foods that one considers healthy, is a relatively new term. It was coined in 1997 by Dr Steven Bratman, an American alternative medicine practitioner, in an essay in the non-scientific *Yoga Journal*. Although orthorexia, also known as orthorexia nervosa, is not currently recognised as an eating disorder in a clinical setting, awareness is on the rise, so this may change in the future.

Orthorexia isn't just about obsessively eating 'healthy' foods, it also has a strong connection with compulsively exercising, in the same way that anorexia and exercise addiction are connected. Eating nutritious foods and getting regular exercise are, of course, fantastic ways to improve your physical and mental wellbeing. However, even healthy behaviours can become problematic when taken to the extreme. At least 39 per cent of people with eating disorders exercise compulsively as well. According to one study, 30 per cent of athletes exhibit symptoms of orthorexia.

Some people with this condition are overly concerned with their appearance, but that is not the case for everyone. It often stems from a need for control, or it can be a way of coping with stress.

My struggles with orthorexia

I want to share my own story here in case it helps others, as in the past, I have suffered with elements of orthorexia. I particularly agonised over the risks and benefits of certain foods and compulsively checked labels on jars and packets. Some days, my inability to decide on the 'best' nutritious meal meant not eating much at all.

I have also been through periods where I was particularly obsessed about numbers and stats. One year it was my blood pressure readings, while at other times I've been transfixed by my weight and body composition. And being a runner, there have been long periods of time where tracking my pace and distance has taken priority. Sometimes, this came at the expense of rest and fully taking care of my body.

Thankfully, my orthorexia and exercise addiction tendencies have usually been short-lived and never severe enough to be formally diagnosed. However, it is something I occasionally still battle with when stress levels become overwhelming, and I feel out of control in other areas of my life. Feeling the need to always be in control can be an issue for me, but I'm working on it.

Studying nutrition for four years was a huge eye-opener for me regarding how each of us has a unique relationship with the food and exercise choices we make, which often stems from childhood learnings and experiences. There is so much conflicting information out there, and an increasing amount of pressure to be, live or look a certain way. My studies highlighted how what – and why – the things we eat, drink and do have the capacity to help or heal us.

Signs and symptoms of orthorexia

Maybe you are wondering whether your own interest in running and healthy eating has become a touch too fanatical. To assess this, there are some general signs and symptoms that are telling. You don't have to display all the signs to be considered ill. Equally, showing one symptom alone does not mean there is anything wrong with you.

Orthorexia symptoms include:

» An obsession with eating foods that one considers healthy.

» Complete avoidance of foods viewed as 'unhealthy'.

» Concern over the risks and benefits of foods and ingredients.

» Cutting out foods, or groups of foods, such as sugar, carbohydrates, dairy and meat.

» Compulsively checking labels or what other people are eating.

» Spending an excessive amount of time thinking about and researching food.

» Experiencing anxiety and stress when desired foods are unavailable.

» Feeling guilt or shame when you stray from your perfect diet.

» Feeling 'in control' when you stick to your planned, healthy diet.

» Judgement of other people's food choices, especially if you view them as less healthy than your own.

If you suspect you may have an eating disorder of any kind, I urge you to talk with a trusted friend or family member and seek help from your GP or an appropriate health professional. Additionally, Beat, the UK's leading charity supporting those affected by eating disorders, offer some great advice and guidance on their website. Find them at www.beateatingdisorders.org.uk.

How orthorexia affects running performance

The negative effects of obsessive healthy eating and dietary restrictions can be dramatic. Cutting out food groups such as dairy for a long period of time can result in reduced bone mass, which for runners immediately increases their risk of injury, especially stress fractures. There is more about this on page 163.

Slowed heart rate and other heart complications can also arise after a prolonged period of restricted eating. Cutting down on the variety of foods you eat on a regular basis reduces the array and possibly the amount of nutrients that go into your body. Nutrient deficiencies impact running performance, recovery and a healthy functioning body in many ways.

Nutrient	Impact of insufficiency
Iron	Iron-deficiency anaemia, which can result in low energy.
Zinc	Compromised immune function, resulting in more frequent and longer-lasting colds and infections.
Calcium	Reduced bone density that increases your risk of injury.
Magnesium	Reduced bone density and poor sleep, which increases your risk of injury.

Bear in mind that if you are training for an endurance event such as a marathon, your body's nutrient requirements will be even higher than before.

How to achieve a more stable relationship with food

Firstly, let me reiterate that if you are in any way concerned that your thoughts and feelings about food and exercise are excessive or overly obsessive, you must seek professional advice from a qualified medical practitioner.

Secondly, enlist help. Sometimes, simply chatting with a fellow runner, friend or partner can open up the conversation and make you feel more supported. Some nutrition practitioners, like myself, are trained to support emotional eating concerns through positive coping skills, education and planning better alternatives. An up-to-date list of registered nutrition practitioners can be found at www. bant.org.uk.

Thirdly, try eating more intuitively, which I appreciate takes a little bit of practice. Intuitive eating means thinking more about what your body needs rather than what you feel you should be eating. One example could be by honouring your hunger after a long run. If you want extra toast and a slice or two of bacon with your eggs, then go for it. If that meal leaves you feeling overly full then make a mental note for next time, but accept the choice you made. It is not helpful to berate yourself for making the 'wrong' food choice.

Get to know your hunger by using a scale rating. For example, one simple saying can be: "On a scale of 1 to 10, I am feeling _ hungry right now."

> Becoming more in tune with your body can be of great benefit to runners, through both food and exercise.

You may benefit from being more careful with the words you use when talking about food choices, both to yourself and out loud. For example:

- ✓ You could replace, "I must not eat bread today" with, "I choose not to eat bread today."

- ✓ You could reframe, "I better have the chicken salad for lunch" with, "Today I choose to have a delicious chicken salad, with dressing on the side for a flavour boost."

The words you use in relation to food have a powerful role to play and the potential to make a positive difference to your relationship with it.

Positive nutrition really does play an important part in recovery from orthorexia. Healthy eating is not something to be feared or followed strictly. A realistic 90/10 balance can work well. That is choosing healthy, balanced meals and good nutrition for 90 per cent of the time, while for the remaining 10 per cent eating exactly what you fancy. By nurturing a healthy relationship with food and drink alongside a balanced relationship with exercise, you will be well on your way to feeling great and running strong.

SECTION 2

TRAINING

Each and every one of you reading this book will be at a different stage of your running journey. Some of you will be just starting out, or you may have been running consistently for 20 years or more. Most of you, I suspect, will be somewhere in between.

This section is all about essential female nutrition for specific running distances, because what you are best off eating when training for your first 10km event is quite different to the food you need when taking part in a 100km ultramarathon over 2 days.

I have split the information up into three parts: shorter distances, including interval and hill training, 10km through to half marathon distances, and marathons and beyond.

CHAPTER 6

SHORTER DISTANCES

For the purposes of this book, 'shorter' means anything up to a 10km distance. Now, I do appreciate that for some of you, running 5km is an awfully long way and 10km is a distance you have only ever dreamed about. I do not mean to belittle your achievements or goals, but for nutrition related to running performance, you have slightly different needs up to the 10km distance than when you run for longer. I want to make it clear, though, that by focusing on and nailing down the right nutrition for you, you will become a stronger runner full stop. This is regardless of what distances you usually run and where you are right now in your training plan.

Building up to 5km

It's awesome when anyone starts running for the very first time, whatever age or stage of life they're at. Some people in the running community either forget or have never experienced how much energy, determination and discomfort it can take to progress from barely being able to run for a bus to running three whole miles in one go.

I'll admit that in the past, I've not really given a second thought to the challenge of building up to a 5km continuous run, because it has been so long since I've had to do that. But twice I have been that 'new' runner. Eleven weeks after my daughter was born, I slowly took some tentative steps back to running, and will never forget the first slow, uncomfortable plod around the block. Five weeks after that, I ran a 4km cross country race (not fast) with a friend and was elated to finish in one piece!

I also remember those early weeks of training, after my surgeon and physio gave me the go ahead to run again after foot surgery mid-2020. The first walk/run felt amazing, but the second time I headed out, this time for a 1-mile run, it was so, so tough. It was like my body had forgotten how! Thankfully, it didn't take long for it to remember again and soon I was happily and comfortably running 5km once again. If you are on the Couch to 5km journey, whatever your starting point, be super proud of yourself. Don't stop believing!

Nutrition for building up to 5km continuous running

In terms of what is best to eat and drink when you are at the beginning of your running story, the simplest and easiest way of taking a step forward is to start with the basics and make small changes to your diet. These should be realistic and sustainable, such as eating fresh fruit and vegetables every day, switching from white to wholemeal bread and increasing your daily water intake. At this stage, you don't need to be concerned with energy gels, beetroot shots or recovery drinks!

I suggest that you refer back to Chapter 1 for a bit about Couch to 5km overeating and the myth that once you start running any distance, you need to be eating carbs morning, noon and night. This is completely unnecessary and, as explained in earlier chapters, focusing purely on carbohydrate foods could be detrimental to your health and running performance.

One of my top pieces of advice is to monitor your food intake to avoid overeating. It is true that running can increase the production of certain hormones that stimulate or suppress the appetite, so keeping track of what and when you eat is useful. As you get into your running stride, you may start to feel hungrier, so base any increase in food intake around healthy choices such as lean meat, complex carbohydrates and vegetables rather than cake.

Dietary basics

Water

Aim to drink at least 6 to 8 glasses over the course of a day, taken at regular intervals. If you are running in warmer weather, you will need to drink even more. Regardless of what time of the day you usually run, drink a glass of water when you wake up in the morning, as you dehydrate naturally overnight. Adding a squeeze of lemon to slightly warm water is a great way to start the day, as it will get your digestive system gently working.

Fresh vegetables and fruits

Aim for 5 portions a day of different vegetables as a minimum to get started, plus 1 or 2 portions of fruit. These are achievable quantities. You can work up gradually to up to 10 portions of veg a day, but when you are starting off on a health journey, keep your goals small and achievable, just like you would with your training. Aim for a variety of veg across any given week. Try and think outside of the carrots and broccoli box!

Quality protein foods

Aim for a portion or two at every meal, plus snacks. Foods like fish, eggs, lean meat, beans, nuts and pulses all count as a portion of protein. Because protein is essential for the growth and repair of your body, it is a vital component of a runner's diet. When you start running, your body needs the right foods to recover effectively and prepare you for the next training run. Some people find the midweek breakfast the most difficult meal to get a portion of protein in. Eggs are a classic choice, but if you are really pushed for time, I suggest boosting up a bowl of porridge with nuts and seeds. Or why not try a simple smoothie to start your day? Here's one I make on a regular basis.

Plant-based, high-protein smoothie:

- » 1 ripe banana, peeled
- » 2 tbsp ground flax seeds
- » 1 tbsp chia seeds
- » 1 tbsp raw cacao powder
- » 50g oats
- » 2 tbsp peanut butter (or cashew or almond butter)
- » 500ml unsweetened almond milk

Blend together the following ingredients to make a generous portion of this plant-based, high-protein smoothie.

Complex carbohydrates

Check back to Chapter 2 for the lowdown on carbohydrate foods for runners and Chapter 1 for why carb loading is not a good idea at this stage. Focus on sensible, moderate portions of complex carbohydrates. You can use your hand as a guide – one cupped handful is a rough portion size. Good food choices include oats, wholegrain rice, potatoes and seeded wholemeal bread. What you want to avoid is refined, white carbs such as white bread and pasta, pastry and the processed carbohydrates found in sweetened breakfast cereals.

Healthy fats

These are essential for all women, as they help with your hormone function, the absorption of fat-soluble vitamins and giving you the necessary energy to run. Fats to focus on include olive oil, avocado, flaxseed, nuts and seeds. Be mindful of your portion size. A small amount of good quality extra virgin olive oil, for example, is a healthier choice than a large quantity of refined sunflower oil.

Minimise unnecessary sugars and processed foods. I am not saying that right now you must cut out every single bit of sugar from your diet, but simply reducing how much you eat is a great start. Trust me, you will feel better for doing that. The energy you gain will go a long way towards helping you achieve your 5km goal.

Keep things simple. At this stage (or arguably any stage of your running journey), you do not need to invest in expensive supplements or fancy foods. When you start out, it's best to focus on whole foods like the ones already mentioned.

How to get the timing of food and running right

New runners frequently ask me about the best time to eat. They want to know whether they should eat breakfast before a morning run or what time to have dinner when some post-work training is on the agenda. There is no one set answer to this, as some runners have stomachs of steel and others need a full three hours to digest a meal before heading out. So, in the beginning, trial and error is your friend. I suggest that you give different timings and foods a go, keep a note of how well they work and adjust your schedule and meal plan accordingly.

To begin with, however, there are some good practices to adopt that will suit most runners.

Best practices

✓ Leave two hours from the time you finish eating a meal to the time you head out of the door for a run. Use the two-hour rule as a starting point and monitor how you feel. You may find that 1.5 hours is fine after breakfast, but three hours feels better later in the day. I've found that I cannot eat either eggs or peanut butter less than 2 hours before going for even a short run, yet other foods are usually fine.

✓ Choose easily digestible foods for your pre-run meal. You don't want anything too high in fat, fibre or protein, as your body takes more effort and a longer time to digest these than simple carbohydrate foods. In particular, watch out for broccoli and other high fibre veg, spicy foods, beans and pulses and caffeine. Instead try oats, bread, sweet potato, pasta and rice. These staple carbohydrate foods will fuel you comfortably through a run.

✓ You may benefit from enjoying a snack 30 minutes to an hour before running. Bananas are a runner's favourite, as they are generally easy on the stomach and have the added benefit of being portable, as they come in their own natural packaging. This is ideal if you need a snack on your commute home from work. Something like a couple of oatcakes spread with honey or marmite before running can work too.

✓ Avoid heavy, fatty foods like sausages and rich sauces that can sit in your stomach for hours. Be careful about eating large portions of any meal, even seemingly healthy foods, because it may take your stomach too long to digest everything comfortably. Many female runners find eating meat, especially red meat like lamb or beef, takes a lot of digesting and, therefore, is not ideal to fill up on in the few hours before running. It is far better to keep meaty, rich meals for afterwards, when the body is in a more relaxed state ready to digest and repair.

✓ Drink some water an hour before you go for a run. Not too much or you'll be needing the loo. Always remember that no matter what the weather is like (yes, even on a cold, wintry day in the UK), it's imperative to run and exercise when well hydrated.

Follow these guidelines and you'll be off to a flying start with your nutrition. Keep track of what you eat, when you eat it and the training you do to pinpoint exactly what foods work best for you. Then you'll be well on your way to a successful 5km run, and perhaps even a longer one.

Parkrun

A Parkrun is 5km in distance and the most common end goal of a Couch to 5km-type programme. If you are a new runner, imagine the elation of your first time running continually for 5km without stopping. It is a feeling like no other. Yes, after reaching the finish line you may be knackered, hot and sweaty (possibly with jelly legs, too), but the sense of accomplishment will put a beaming smile on your face.

Thousands of men and women around the world spend their Saturday mornings in parks and cities running or walking 5km around carefully mapped-out routes with hundreds of other people. The events provide a wonderful, free community for runners, no matter what their age or ability. It's well worth looking up.

The step up from training to running your first 5km is more about the regularity of running than increasing the distance you go, at least initially. Ideally, this goes hand in hand with the regularity of eating healthy, balanced meals, meaning it's a great time to get to grips with specific foods that do and do not suit you, plus the all-important meal timings.

Nutrition and lifestyle for your best Parkrun

First off, there isn't usually a need to load up with carbohydrates before – or fuel up during – a Parkrun. This rule applies whatever level you're at. What you do, eat and drink on the evening before the run is arguably the most important thing.

A good night's sleep is useful so that ideally you wake up feeling refreshed. Having a solid, balanced meal comprising a portion of carbohydrates, some fresh veg and a portion of protein is best to have the evening before you head out. There should be nothing too fatty, spicy or unusual in your meal that could either cause digestive problems or give you a poor night's sleep.

On the Friday before Parkrun, it's best to skip the alcohol. I totally get that you may want to celebrate the start of the weekend, but indulging in a tipple or two is best saved until Saturday night, unless, of course, you are planning a Sunday run too. Instead, hydrate with plain water and perhaps use this time as an opportunity to try out the plethora of alcohol-free drinks that are now available. My personal favourite Friday night drink is kombucha, a fizzy, fermented green tea drink that comes in a whole host of flavours. Served in a champagne glass, it can almost be mistaken for a real glass of fizz. Kombucha is infinitely healthier and more likely to help you run a great 5km on Saturday morning.

Alcohol-free drinks:

- » Sparkling water and a slice of lemon
- » Kombucha
- » Herbal tea – there are many flavours available to try
- » Ginger beer
- » Alcohol-free gin and tonic

You want to arrive at the starting line feeling rested and calm, with just a little bit of nervous energy to power you up for a great beginning.

The day before Parkrun, spend some time thinking about the practicalities of which kit you intend to wear and the logistics of how to get to the start of the race, as you'll want to feel calm before you start. Don't do what I've often done when travelling to a new Parkrun and leave too late, only to have difficulty finding parking. More than once, I've literally raced to the start line and then continued running, as the whistle had already gone.

Try your best to arrive feeling relaxed. Not only will it help you to run a smoother and stronger race, but your stomach will thank you for it. Stress and anxiety can easily contribute to an upset stomach that either makes you urgently need the bathroom or clogs you up, leaving you feeling heavy and bloated. Neither are conducive to an enjoyable Parkrun. So, try to minimise stress beforehand and get organised.

Should I eat breakfast before Parkrun?

This is one of those questions without a straightforward 'yes' or 'no' answer. You may be able to run fasted, which means running before eating, but this doesn't suit everyone. Personally, a fasted Parkrun is an absolute 'no' for me because it starts too late. By the time 9am rolls around, I've usually been awake for almost three hours (yes, even at weekends I often wake up shortly after 6am) and my stomach is well and truly awake and calling for food. Running fasted is easier if you literally wake up, roll out of bed and run out of the door.

As with everything nutrition related, what works for me may not work for you. This is the beauty of being an individual.

5 breakfast options before a Parkrun

1. **Porridge.** If eaten 90 to 120 minutes before Parkrun, porridge will give you all the energy you need. Add some raisins or banana and a drizzle of honey and you'll up your energy levels even more. Oats are a slow-release form of complex carbohydrate, meaning they do not spike your blood sugars, but instead give you sustained energy that releases gradually. This is perfect for a short, sharp 5km run. Top tip: to avoid stomach issues, use the type of milk that suits you best or stick with plain water.

2. **Pancakes.** You need not miss out on weekend pancakes. With a little planning, they can make a great breakfast to fuel you to a Parkrun PB. It is best to avoid refined white flour as a pancake base. Instead, try using buckwheat flour to maximise the nutritional value. Despite its name, buckwheat is gluten-free and, therefore, suitable for those with Coeliac disease and anyone sensitive to gluten. If you prepare a simple batter the night before and store it in the fridge overnight, you'll be ready to go first thing Saturday morning. A simple batter recipe I love is: 100g buckwheat flour, 300ml milk (whichever type you favour), 1 egg. Once cooked, buckwheat pancakes can be topped with warm berries, honey and/or nut butter, or eat them plain on the go,

3. **Banana and coffee.** If you are the kind of person who has a late Friday night and then just wants to roll out of bed and go straight out of the door come Saturday morning, then the first two breakfast options may not work so well for you. You need something mega quick and easy to grab as you get your running kit on. A banana will fill you up and provide some energy, with the added benefit of being rich in potassium and magnesium, which are vital minerals for runners. Coffee has been shown to improve running performance in some athletes, though it is by no means suitable for everyone. Read on to the section on 10km training for more information about the pros and cons of caffeine for runners. The key thing with any pre-Parkrun breakfast option is timing. Banana and coffee provide a sharp energy boost that will be quick to take effect, so timing is key. Having them something like half an hour to 45 minutes before starting to run may work best.

4. **Bagel and nut butter.** Here's a classic example of what suits one runner not necessarily suiting another. Many years ago, I did a 5km time trial a couple of hours after eating peanut butter on toast. Let's just say my stomach was not impressed. It was a horrific run and I still shudder at the memory. However, other runners swear by nut butters to fuel them through morning runs. Bagels, especially if you choose wholemeal versions, provide great energy from the carbohydrates they contain. Nut butters are packed full of protein and vital vitamins and minerals. As with porridge, they are best eaten 90 to 120 minutes before running, to allow time for digestion.

5. **Breakfast/snack bar.** Breakfast bars, oat bars, granola bars, or whatever you prefer to call them, are portable, oat-based snacks with added extras like dried fruit. Watch out, though, because these bars tend to be loaded with sugar, so they are not an everyday healthy food choice. However, eaten an hour before Parkrun, these types of bars can be useful to give your body the energy boost it needs in order to nail your run. The combination of oats provides slow-release energy and the dried fruit and sugar give an instant boost that is exactly

what you need right before the race starts. You want to go for something that is higher in carbs and lower in fibre and fat, so it's easy to digest and process into fuel for your body. Protein bars are higher in protein and fat, so they are more suited for eating after the run, when your muscles need to recover.

Whether you eat before Parkrun or not, you must drink water before heading off, and this is regardless of what the weather is like or how quickly you plan to finish. As soon as you wake, I suggest that you drink a large glass of water to rehydrate, and then sip another 300-500ml in the hour before the run starts.

Don't be tempted to down a large bottle of water right before the race starts, as too much liquid jiggling around in your stomach feels wholly unpleasant when moving. My top tip is to use the toilet facilities right before the run starts, whether you think you need them or not.

If you do choose to run a Parkrun, or another 5km, fasted, then make sure you eat soon after finishing. In order to recover properly, your body will need to quickly refuel and reenergise. This is where protein shakes and energy bars come in handy. They are convenient forms of replenishment to leave in your car or kit bag, which you can snack on before heading home for a well-deserved shower and big breakfast.

Hill and interval training

Simply put, hill training involves running up and down hills, often the same one several times! There is no getting around the fact that this is tougher than running on a flat surface, but the benefits are huge. Training consistently on hills makes you a stronger runner by improving both the strength and endurance of your leg muscles, your VO2 max and your resting heart rate. You'll also gain faster speeds on the flat. What's not to like?

As well as more traditional hill training, which involves repeatedly running hard up a hill before recovering by walking or jogging back down it again, you can also incorporate it into a longer run by choosing a route that takes in several hills. If you run up them rather than walking, you'll gain the same benefits.

Interval training involves a series of high intensity runs interspersed with periods of low intensity ones. Put simply, intervals are when you run at different speeds and intensities for a specific number of minutes. The rationale behind it is that it increases running speed and endurance in a limited amount of time. This type of training has been shown to quickly improve oxygen absorption and cardiovascular fitness, so if you have a lot on, it could be perfect for you. Here's a quick word of warning, though, interval training might be shorter in duration, but it is by no means easy. Just like hill training, it is tough on your body, so it's not something you want to be doing every day. The general rule is to leave two or three days between a long run and interval or hill training, which will allow your body sufficient time to recover.

Benefits of hills and intervals for female runners

There is good news for female runners. New research shows that when it comes to running, they may get more out of high intensity interval training than their male counterparts. The study found meaningful differences in the way men and women self-regulate during workouts. During the high-intensity intervals, the women tended to work 'harder' than the men, which was shown through the cardiovascular markers %HRmax and %VO2max. Fundamentally, the women in the research study paid more attention to how they were feeling and were better able to listen to and trust their bodies. Thus, they gained more speed and endurance benefits.

Nutrition for hill and interval training

As I have already said, both hill and interval-type running training are tough on your body, as they increase your heart rate quicker and to a higher level than running on the flat. Because of this, the risk of feeling sick while training is increased, as blood flow is quickly redirected from your stomach to your hard-working muscles. If you still have undigested food in your stomach, it will remain there for the duration of your run, which could make you feel nauseous.

Leave a gap of 2 to 3 hours between eating and heading out for a training session. How quickly food is digested is different for everyone and it also depends on what you eat, so my best advice is to experiment and keep a log of what works and what doesn't. A few studies suggest that female runners benefit from a longer gap between eating and running than men do, but again, it really is down to the individual. Personally, I need three hours after a meal before I'm able to run a decent interval training session or some hill reps without feeling queasy. I have found that even a small snack in the few hours before intense training often doesn't work well for my stomach. The only thing that seems OK is a spoonful of honey, which I use for an instant carbohydrate boost.

To run at speed, you do need sufficient fuel and glycogen stores in your muscles. Think about it this way: if you are interval training at 7pm and lunch was at midday, the energy obtained from the said lunch is unlikely to be enough to see you through an intense session. In this situation, a 4pm snack could come in very handy.

The aim is to choose foods that will provide you with the necessary sustained energy for your training session and that you will also tolerate and digest easily.

Meal ideas before interval training:

- ✓ A jacket potato with tuna or beans and a little bit of butter.
- ✓ Chicken wraps with some salad.
- ✓ A bowl of granola, natural yoghurt and berries.

What these meals have in common is that they contain a combination of carbohydrates, with some protein and a little bit of dietary fat.

EAT WELL, RUN STRONG – HELEN MORTON

They are also relatively 'plain' foods, making them more likely to be digested and tolerated prior to intense running.

Hill and interval running rely mainly on glucose as fuel, so the carbohydrate part of the meal is the most important. Without sufficient carbs, you may well struggle through the session. Just bear in mind that these are meal ideas and not a prescriptive meal plan. As you now know, the food and training that suits you best is unique to you.

Don't be afraid to try different foods out, and when you hit upon a great meal and suitable timeframe that gives you loads of energy for a training session, write it down and remember it for next time.

Hydration for hill and interval training

As I have already explained, hill training elevates your heart rate like nothing else, and as a result you'll sweat more (whatever the weather). Hence, in order to avoid feeling lethargic or dizzy, it's crucial to begin a hill training session fully hydrated. The session is likely to involve hard exertion – running up hills is never easy – so you'll need to have some water with you. Sip rather than guzzle it, or you'll run the risk of that horrible feeling of water sloshing around in your stomach, which could make you feel sick. Sipping water on a regular basis is sufficient to meet your general hydration needs. But if you are running for over an hour, sweat a lot or it is an extremely hot day, then an electrolyte drink may be more beneficial.

Caffeine

Caffeine is the world's most widely used drug, perhaps surprisingly surpassing even nicotine and alcohol. Chemically, it is similar to the drugs morphine and codeine, and just like its chemical counterparts, it can be highly addictive. Up to a certain point, caffeine is a legal performance-enhancing drug (also called an ergogenic aid), but the International Olympic Committee (IOC) has imposed limits on all athletes, showing just how much it affects our bodies.

Many studies exalt the benefits of recreational runners drinking coffee before heading out, linking caffeine intake to improved endurance and speed. It is thought that caffeine boosts blood-adrenaline levels while increasing anaerobic (oxygen-independent) energy production. An increase in adrenaline stimulates more calcium to rush inside muscle cells during contractions, boosting their strength and power. This rise in anaerobic energy production can enable runners to exercise at high intensities for longer periods of time. These two reasons alone mean that a cup of coffee or a caffeine shot or gel can be ideal to take just before hill reps or interval training.

However, I believe there can be some dangers in drinking coffee before an intense run. Let me explain. The adrenaline-like effect that it can produce gives your body a huge boost, causing you to stand up and fight or run away. This increases your heart rate, anxiety and irritable emotions, which on their own wouldn't necessarily be a problem, but if you are already arriving at a club track session or your local park feeling nervous and a little stressed, then an extra adrenaline boost may tip you over the edge. In some runners, the increased heart rate and blood pressure that comes from an extra cup of coffee before embarking on an intense run could be unwise. In certain athletes, caffeine also has the potential to cause diarrhoea. Plus, it is known to interfere with oestrogen production and metabolism. Therefore, it is imperative to weigh up the potential short-term performance-enhancing benefits against the negative impact on your long-term health. Perhaps save the caffeine for when you have an important race and want to be at your peak and putting in a great performance.

Just remember that people have very individualised responses to caffeine.

Here, Dr Eve Pearce of myDNAhealth explains how genetics plays a significant role in how we each deal with caffeine, and why those of you with a low caffeine tolerance could do well to avoid it, no matter how much positive research there is for it enhancing performance.

Genetics of caffeine and running

Caffeine and perceived improved running performance have long been linked. Just a quick internet search will pull up pages of advice and tips. It's even mixed into sports nutrition products such as drinks and gels. But how do we know which of this advice is based on scientific fact? Genomics can give us some key insights.

The CYP1A2 (Cytochrome P-450 1A2) gene produces one of the many enzymes needed for the breakdown of substances that need to be removed from the body (detoxification). A well-known target of CYP1A2 is caffeine, with the majority metabolised by this enzyme. A genetic variation in the CYP1A2 gene is commonly used to identify individuals as either 'fast' or 'slow' metabolisers of caffeine. Interestingly, the benefits of caffeine and exercise have been identified in 'fast' metabolisers only. Research on athletes shows that ingesting moderate amounts of caffeine improves aerobic or muscular endurance-type exercise (such as resistance training and cycling time trials). The overall message here is that moderate caffeine intake before endurance-type running is only beneficial in CYP1A2 'fast' metabolisers. However, it is essential to note that everyone should moderate their caffeine intake. Whilst 'fast' metabolisers can safely have up to two to three cups of coffee a day, 'slow' ones are advised to stick to one, in order to reduce the health risks, such as hypertension.

Recovery nutrition

Recovery from hill training and interval sessions is hugely important, because these types of running are so tough on your leg muscles, particularly your quadriceps, glutes, hamstrings and calves. If you want to run every few days, your muscles need to recover quickly. However, unless you are a competitive elite athlete you do not need to worry too much about immediate nutritional recovery.

It used to be thought that for any benefits to be felt, you must eat within 30 minutes of finishing a run, but that is only true if you are training multiple times a day. For regular runners doing three to five sessions a week, and never more than one run a day, eating within an hour or so after finishing is sufficient for your body to recover and repair effectively.

DOMS (delayed-onset muscle soreness) is common after hill running, which is partly due to the concentric action of the quads on the downhill sections. For many runners, the uphill sections of hill training feel the toughest at the time, while going downhill causes the most aches and pains the day after.

Recovery nutrition for hills and intervals ideally focus on antioxidants to squash the free radicals produced, plus anti-inflammatory foods to regulate inflammatory response and muscle soreness, carbohydrate to replenish glycogen stores and protein for muscular repair. These foods are covered in detail in Chapter 9, but here is a taster of the types of foods that can be useful for recovery from shorter, more intense runs.

The types of foods that can be useful for recovery	
Antioxidants	A wide range of brightly and deeply coloured fruits and vegetables, herbs and spices and green tea.
Anti-inflammatory foods	Oily fish, flaxseed oil, walnuts, olive oil and green, leafy vegetables.
Carbohydrates	Fresh vegetables and fruits, whole grains, beans and pulses.
Proteins	Lean meat, poultry, eggs, pulses and tofu.

CHAPTER 7

10 KM AND UP

Now let's move onto training nutrition for longer distances of 10km through to a half marathon (21km or 13.1 miles). This is where nutrition gets a little more serious.

10km

For some of you, running 10km might be no more than a dream at present, while for others it will be barely worth breaking a sweat for. Wherever you are on the scale, running this kind of distance is where putting a little more thought into nutrition can pay dividends.

Ten-kilometre races can feel tough because they are speedier than a half marathon, but at the same time they are twice as long as a 5km Parkrun. Personally, I love a 10km race. Although it takes me 10 minutes or so to get into a good rhythm and settle down to the pace I want, once I'm there I'm sorted for the rest of the race; 5km is over with too quickly, so my poor old legs don't get the chance to get into a proper tempo before it's time to stop! Regardless of whether 10km is a distance you enjoy or one you are working towards running in the future, getting into the right mindset about the training, pacing and fuelling is important in making the distance a success.

Nutrition for 10km running

Timing of food and what to eat

When it comes to what time you eat before a 10km race, it's no different to any other distance. It's all about maximising energy from food and minimising digestive problems like bloating, sickness or heartburn.

Eating some breakfast around two hours before starting a morning run of a 45-90-minute duration works for many women. Two hours gives enough time for the food to be fully digested and for all the useful nutrients to be absorbed, yet it is not so far in advance that you'll feel hungry again. Most runners find that this timeframe gives them the best of both worlds.

Complex carbohydrates, as explained in Chapter 2, provide sustaining energy in the form of muscle glycogen and should form the basis of any pre-run meal.

Oats are a great staple carbohydrate food that many runners rely on. The complex carbohydrate that oats are made from are slowly released into the bloodstream, giving a sustained level of energy rather than an instant boost that quickly fades. Oats can take the form of oatcakes, which are perfect spread with a little honey, for a no-cook breakfast, traditional porridge or newer and trendier 'overnight' oats. If you have not come across the concept of overnight oats before, they are a no-cook version of porridge. Raw oats are soaked with milk, water or juice, allowing the oats to absorb the liquid and soften them enough to eat uncooked. Keep them in the fridge overnight (hence the name) and they'll be ready to go in the morning. If you are a fan of running early, then overnight oats can be a godsend.

The breakfast options for a Parkrun on page 127 all hold true for 10km running, as they contain complex carbohydrates to give your body the energy it needs. Toast or cereal are common breakfast choices for many female runners. There is nothing wrong with these, I would just recommend that you choose the wholegrain versions, such as wholemeal bread, low-sugar muesli or granola, or shredded wheat.

CHAPTER SEVEN – 10KM AND UP

Protein and dietary fat are not necessary in the few hours before running, and certainly not for the 10km distance, although they still need to be included as part of your daily diet. A lot of runners find that eating fatty foods makes them feel a little queasy, especially if they are eaten right before running. Having said that, I do know some runners who thrive on bacon and eggs before a race. The joys of individuality.

What about if you are running later in the day, for example, after work?

The same nutritional rules apply. Try and eat a carbohydrate-rich meal or snack around two hours before starting your run. For example, if you are intending to run at 5pm and lunch was at 1pm, you would benefit from topping up your glycogen stores with a small snack at around 3pm. If you choose some easily digestible carbohydrate, like a banana, some trail mix or an oat bar, your muscles should have sufficient energy to run 10km well.

Fuelling during a 10km run

Do you need to take on fuel during a 10km run? Probably not, but if it is an important race or you know that the route is an exceptionally hilly one and will take longer than it might usually do, or even if you just feel like you need a boost, then take on some carbohydrate fuel, such as an energy gel, during the run. I suggest that you experiment with the timing of taking them, as some people feel the effects within a few minutes, while for others it takes 15 minutes or so for the energy boost to kick in. There's more about this in the section on marathon running on page 150.

Hydration for 10km running

Sufficient hydration is vital for strong running. When you are running for 60 minutes and more, which many of you will be doing on a 10km run, you will benefit from carrying some water to sip. How much fluid you choose to drink during the run is your call, but having the option at least will put your mind at rest, especially as the run progresses and you find that you are working harder and sweating more. Use your own judgement, depending on how you are feeling, the intensity of the run and the weather. On a cold, wintry day in the UK, you probably won't feel like you need to drink as much water as you would on a summer's day, but even sipping a little bit can refresh your mind and body and give you a well-needed boost.

Remember that thirst is a poor indicator of hydration, because by the time you feel thirsty you could already be dehydrated. The general rule of thumb is to drink water while running before you feel like you need it.

I have covered what is best to eat and drink before, during and after running 10km. Essentially, think of it as a step up from 5km nutrition, and just as you would with your training, make a few adjustments here and there. Keep your day-to-day nutrition basics, including regular balanced meals, snacks and water, in place by eating enough and eating well. Add in some recovery foods and possibly some extra fuelling before and during a run. These simple things will set you off on a great path to strong, consistent 10km running.

Recovery nutrition

As with hill and interval training, nutrition once you have finished running is all about the recovery. You need to refuel by replenishing glycogen stores and repairing your muscles ready to run again within whatever timeframe you have set.

As such, a meal high in carbohydrate, protein and antioxidants is your basic go-to. Just bear in mind that no matter how hungry you may feel straight after running (some women find their appetite increases while for others it diminishes), there is no need to eat in excess. Unless you are particularly looking to gain weight, keep portion sizes moderate.

Fasted running

As already discussed, anecdotal research says that most women find running a 10km distance easier if they have eaten something a few hours beforehand. However, there are always exceptions to the rule, and many women run better fasted. Often it depends on how long you have been running for, because after several years of consistent running training, it is perfectly normal for your body to adapt. Please note that although some of you, myself included, will run well before breakfast, if you are just starting to move up from 5km to 10km then do not expect this strategy to work straightaway, as it can take a bit of getting used to.

In simple terms, fasted running is when you run after a long stretch without eating, most commonly in the morning before breakfast. You literally wake up, drink a glass of water and go.

Training in a depleted state has been well-researched, in both male and female runners. Although there are some benefits to fasted running training, there are also downsides and potential risks, especially for women. It may work for you or it may not. Our physiology is fascinating because it is so highly variable.

Some studies suggest that fasted training could possibly increase the capacity for the body to oxidate fat to fuel running, also known as fat-adapted. The theory is that by improving fat oxidation, even just a little, a runner can move faster for longer by pushing closer to their limit right from the start. Occasional fasted runs may be useful for some women, but I would argue that they are not something to be done every single time you go for a run.

Despite the performance benefits of fasted running training that some studies report, the risks other multiple studies have found include reduced performance due to low energy availability. Practice in running fasted can reduce the negative impact on performance, but overall, it is still likely to undermine peak performance, except possibly during low-intensity, easy runs.

Half marathon

Nutrition for a half marathon is sometimes overlooked, but, in my view, you put in a lot of training, so why not give your nutrition the same respect? It could make all the difference in running your best half.

Even if you don't intend to race this distance, every time you run upwards of 10 miles you want to be thinking about what you eat and drink, both before and after training. For me, a leisurely Sunday morning 10 to 13 miler over local hilly trails with a friend or my run club group could mean running for 2 to 3 hours. That much time on my feet means that fuelling during the run is necessary.

Nutrition for half marathon running

Timing of food and what to eat

Ideally, you want to be eating around two hours before a run, in the same way as you would for the 10km distance. Choose a carbohydrate-rich meal that will provide sufficient glucose to ensure that you are starting out with full glycogen stores.

Half marathon runners rely heavily on glucose as fuel, so you need a carbohydrate-dominant diet. This does not mean consuming a carbohydrate-only diet; protein and dietary fat are still important macronutrients for all runners.

You may find that a combination of glucose and fructose gives the best sustained energy, as once consumed, fructose kicks in at a slower rate than glucose. In practice, this could mean having a banana on toast, some pasta with passata sauce or overnight oats topped with berries. I always advise experimenting with different meals and snacks to see what works best for you. However, if you are running a half marathon event, whether for the first or seventeenth time, your race day breakfast should be a well-tested meal that you know gives you plenty of energy and no stomach issues. Race day is not the time to be trying out new nutrition strategies.

Some runners find that consuming a gel or a small, glucose-rich snack like half a banana, a spoonful of honey or a couple of dates 15 to 30 minutes before setting off, especially if racing or training at near-race pace, can give an extra boost of glucose and energy that sustains their effort for longer. Again, this is something to try out yourself and see how much, if any, benefit it produces.

Note: Fasted running is not recommended for this type of distance, unless you are well trained and have a specific reason for doing so.

Before a longer run, such as a half marathon, it is useful to ensure that you are well rested, though I appreciate that in practice this may not always be possible. We all experience stress from time to time, which can deplete vital stores of micronutrients such as zinc, iron, vitamin B6 and magnesium. Ideally, as well as consuming regular carbohydrate-rich foods to ensure muscle glycogen stores are topped up, also incorporate a range of fresh vegetables, fruits, beans, pulses, meat, fish, eggs, nuts and seeds into your daily diet. This will maximise your intake of vitamins and minerals. Drinking water regularly in the day before a longer run is also important to ensure you start your run fully hydrated.

Beetroot juice

Beetroot juice has been well studied in recent years as an aid for faster running and better stamina. Most studies concur that one to two shots of concentrated beetroot juice taken two to three hours before exercise can be of benefit, but the biggest gains seem to come from drinking it every day for the week building up to a half marathon race. Research has also found that the benefits of beetroot juice are greater in athletes that haven't trained as much. So, if you are training for your first half marathon it might be worth experimenting with some beetroot shots.

So, what is so special about beetroot? Well, it is a rich source of potent antioxidants, including vitamin C, carotenoids, phenolic acids and flavonoids, along with being rich in nitrates. Once ingested, the body converts nitrates to nitric oxide, which is known to enhance blood vessel dilation and increase the delivery of oxygen and nutrients to working muscles during exercise, thus helping to increase running speeds. Research suggests that blood nitric oxide levels peak 2 to 3 hours after ingestion and approach the baseline 12 hours later, so allow a few hours for the beetroot to take effect.

Rather than cooking up a whole pile of beetroot for lunch, beetroot shots of concentrated juice are a more convenient way of gaining performance benefits. Shots typically contain 400mg of dietary nitrates in a 70ml bottle, which is equivalent to 500ml of beetroot juice. I know which I would rather drink!

Fuelling during a half marathon

When running training increases in time and you start doing longer runs of over 90 minutes, taking on fuel during the run becomes more important, especially during an intense run at or near to race pace. If a half marathon is a step towards your first marathon, then use this training period to test out different fuelling strategies for the big day. You may be able to make it through a half marathon in reasonable shape with less-than-ideal fuelling, but a full marathon is a different story. Take this time to practise and try out different approaches.

Carbohydrate intake is most important, as it is rapidly and easily converted to glucose to supply working muscles with sufficient energy to maintain high-intensity running. Do refer back to Chapter 2, Nutrition Basics, for in-depth information about carbohydrates.

Many runners start to experiment with energy gels during their half marathon training. These are highly concentrated sources of carbohydrates, generally providing 25-30 grams in each tube. This gives your muscles a much-needed boost of energy to keep them running strongly for the full distance. The energy gels market is an extremely competitive and quickly evolving one, and it's a whole different ball game to when I first started running in 1996, when there were only a few options available. The typical old-school energy gels utilise maltodextrin as a carbohydrate source, which many runners find can cause nausea and stomach distress. However, each brand is subtly different, so rest assured there will be at least one out there that will suit you.

Most energy gels are absorbed best when they are taken with a little water, but there are new formulations that rely less on liquid to take effect. For some runners, it's the gooey texture of energy gels that can be the biggest turn-off, as they can be thick and difficult to swallow while gasping for air. Personally, I was put off by the old gloopy gels that needed too much chewing and made me want to gag. Nowadays, there are some delicious-tasting gels with much thinner textures that are a joy to eat. Chewable blocks of jelly and enhanced jellybeans are also available, if that is your preference! Read page 150 for more advice on energy gels and the lowdown on the best options available.

Hydration for half marathon running

As already discussed in Chapter 2, drinking too much plain water during a long run can be detrimental. Ten miles upwards is a good distance to start thinking about using electrolyte drinks or salt tablets. Replenishing salts, the electrolytes that your body needs to function, is vital during longer distance running, particularly during hot and humid weather. You may be able to make it through a 5km to 10km run in one piece without replenishing lost salts, but try that on a hot day for more than 10 miles and you'll risk not only poor performance but also health issues, including cramps, nausea, headaches and even hyponatraemia (a low level of sodium in the blood, causing lethargy and confusion).

Don't be fooled into thinking that you won't need to carry water with you when running in winter. Even in colder weather, you need to drink as you run because the intense exercise will still cause you to gain body heat and sweat. For those runners who wrap up in several layers at the slightest chill in the air, or who run a half marathon in over two hours, hydration is especially important.

Recovery nutrition

The more miles you run the more critical recovery nutrition becomes. The basis of a stronger, more energetic body free from injury comes from regularly breaking down muscle tissue and then consuming the right nutrition afterwards. Recovery nutrition is key in repairing and recovering all the cells of your body.

Immediately after endurance running, the topmost priority is for carbohydrate stores to be replenished. The best snack to eat is one that will get simple carbohydrate into the bloodstream quickly, at the same time as some protein to help speed glycogen production and muscular repair. Something like a couple of rice cakes spread with nut butter, a banana and a handful of almonds, or a specially designed recovery drink can make great choices. If you are aiming to lose weight it is a mistake to think that restricting food straight after running will help. By not eating for several hours after a training session, your body becomes more stressed and fatigue kicks in, making you less able to perform strongly during your next run. Increased cortisol levels cause the body to retain fat and break down muscle tissue, which is the opposite of what you intended.

A snack straight after finishing a long run will get the recovery process started, then, once you are showered and stretched, it's time for a complete meal. Ideally, this will consist of high-quality protein, complex carbohydrates, omega-3 EFAs and a range of vitamins and minerals.

One popular post-running meal is eggs on toast, which I would boost up and make nutrient-dense by using sourdough bread, adding some sautéed mushrooms and grilled tomatoes, a large handful of rocket, a sprinkling of pumpkin seeds and a drizzle of flaxseed oil. Now, THAT is what I call a perfectly balanced post-endurance-run recovery meal.

CHAPTER 8

MARATHON AND BEYOND

These are the big distances, the events that some of you may take on as either a one-off challenge or a step up after the marathon distance. Taking on these kinds of running distances and events is becoming more popular than ever, so it stands to reason that appropriate nutritional strategies are also being investigated. Of course, many of you may skip this section completely, especially if you are just starting on your running journey. This is completely fine, but perhaps keep the book in case you need it for another time. All the information will then be here, ready and waiting for when you need it. And if you never want to run a marathon then that is fine, too. Maybe pass the book on so another runner can read this chapter.

Marathon

The marathon distance is a long way – 26.2 miles (42km) to be exact. For many runners, it will be the furthest you have ever run in one go.

> Do not underestimate the achievement of preparing for and running a marathon.

You have a lot of training to do, which can become all-encompassing. In order to succeed on race day, you need to be purposeful in what you eat and drink and how much you rest during the whole of your training period, and in particular the crucial week before the marathon. And of course, what you eat and drink during the race itself will be a primary focus. You will have put in too many long miles of running and training to give your marathon event up to luck

Nutrition for marathon running

This is where everything you have learned in previous chapters about the basics and myths of running nutrition will stand you in good stead. Unlike with shorter distances, for a marathon and beyond, nutrition becomes a necessary function instead of just an option.

I suggest you put as much thought into what you eat and drink on training days, especially on your long run day, as you will for the race day itself. The training weeks are not only a chance to run many miles and get your legs and mind ready for the full distance, they are also the perfect opportunity to get your nutritional strategy down to a tee.

Marathon training builds up over 16 to 20 weeks, gradually increasing the length of your runs until you are comfortably going upwards of 18 miles. Being purposeful about what you eat and drink and how much rest and recovery you take over the training period will give you the best chance of success, not only on the race day itself but also for continued health and performance gains. Just as you do with running training, I suggest approaching nutrition changes gradually. This way they stand a better chance of becoming long-term lifestyle shifts that will keep you eating well and running strong for years to come.

The food and drink you choose is a fundamental basis of strong running. Go back to Chapter 2 for everything you need to know about what a strong runner's diet needs to include and why. Begin with where your nutrition is right now, which is a great way to work out what changes you need to make. A simple way to do this is by taking the time to write a 7-day food, mood and training diary. This can help to set you off on the right path, by highlighting the foods that are already working for your running and the ones that need adjusting.

Reminder of nutrition strategies for endurance running

✓ Before each run, ensure that you are well fuelled by consuming a meal based around carbohydrates in the few hours before heading out.

✓ Ensure that you stay hydrated every day by drinking 1.5 to 2 litres of water, spread across the day, plus extra water during and after your longer runs.

✓ Eat enough. Many marathon runners find their appetite naturally increases with their mileage, however, in some women, appetite is suppressed, and it can feel like a challenge to eat enough to fuel all the energy expended. Healthy fats and quality protein are calorie-dense foods that should be included in every meal.

The right nutrition is vital in efficiently repairing damaged muscles and recovering ready for your next training run. Consuming simple carbohydrate straight after a run will ensure muscle glycogen stores are quickly restored. Follow this with a meal, ideally containing at least 20g of protein, a rainbow of antioxidant-rich vegetables and some anti-inflammatory omega-3 fatty acids from flaxseed or oily fish.

It takes practice to get your nutrition spot on, and as your training evolves depending on your current goals and life load, your nutritional strategies should always have an element of flexibility.

The week before marathon race day

Ensure that your glycogen stores are maximised by slightly increasing the amount of carbohydrate foods you consume. There is no need to carb load in the old-fashioned way, as explained back in Chapter 1. The combination of slightly increasing your carb intake by eating slightly larger portion sizes and reducing your training to keep your legs feeling fresh and rested will help to maximise glycogen stores in the muscles.

Marathon race day

Most marathon runners do not run the whole 26.2 miles before race day. The event itself is the pinnacle of many months of training. Keep to the same routine as you have for your long training runs. Relax as much as you can. Feeling too anxious can cause an upset stomach.

Fuelling during a marathon is vital, and by now you should know what suits you best. As a reminder, to start with, taking on around 30g of carbohydrate every 45 minutes is a good rule of thumb.

Energy gels

On page 139, I talked about the use of energy gels during a race, for a regular intake of carbohydrates to keep glycogen stores topped up. There are a huge range of options currently available. Here are four that I have personally recently tried.

Energy Gels – how they stack up	
Veloforte	Based on natural ingredients with a range of more interesting flavours, such as date, lemon and ginger, and beetroot and lemon. 22g of carbohydrates in a smaller-than-average 33g serving. It has a pleasant texture and I felt absorption was enhanced when taken with a little water.
SiS GO Isotonic Energy	Easy to find both in shops and online, with a wide range of flavours and a very reasonable price. Each gel provides 22g of carbohydrates. Some also contain caffeine or electrolytes. No need to take them with water. Fairly watery consistency so easy to consume during running, but the taste is a little artificial and unappealing.

Energy Gels – how they stack up	
Mulebar	A wide range of strong flavours available in reusable energy gel pouches, with refill bottles available to cut down on plastic. Made from more natural ingredients, including agave syrup, brown rice syrup and pink Himalayan salt crystals. Each gel provides up to 28g of carbohydrates, depending on the flavour.
33 Fuel Chia energy gel	Fully vegan with just four ingredients, including their trademark chia seeds. Quite different to regular gels in that they arrive in dried form and you prep them yourself by adding a little water. Each gel provides 11.3g of carbohydrates. They provide energy very well, but as I am not a fan of chia seeds, they took some getting used to.

Recovery nutrition

When training for a marathon, recovery nutrition is as important as the training itself, as it helps to stave off injuries and ensure you remain as healthy as possible. Extra lifestyle changes, including plenty of sleep, stretching and downtime are also required. There is no getting around the fact that running these kinds of distances is time-consuming and tiring work.

Some women become overly concerned about their weight when training for a marathon, which is partly because when looking at elite runners, you could be forgiven for thinking that you need to be tiny and stick thin. But runners of all shapes and sizes successfully run marathons. There is, thankfully, no requirement to look like Paula Radcliffe. You are a marathon runner whatever your waistline and weight and regardless of how long it takes you to complete the distance. Besides, under eating is in no way helpful when training for endurance events, since although you may feel lighter and faster after a bit of weight loss, your body could well be lacking essential nutrients and calories for good health, great energy and strong bones, to name just a few.

Focus on Intermittent Fasting

Intermittent fasting (IF) is a nutrition trend that has endured and evolved in recent years to now include a concept called time-restricted feeding (TRF). Both practices are based around a period of time when you do not eat (the fasting period) and a shorter period of time when you are allowed to eat (the feeding period). The 5:2 diet, as made famous by the former doctor and now TV presenter Michael Mosley, is a popular weight-loss method of eating that has much scientific backing, and can lead to significant health improvements and weight reduction. This is just one type of IF, and there are many different variations on the theme.

I could find no strong evidence for IF practices improving endurance running performance, though there is plenty of anecdotal evidence amongst the running community, including when it comes to weight management and increased energy outside of training.

Research does, however, point towards potential downsides to IF, particularly in reduced recovery and muscle growth after intense training, which can impair marathon running potential. Consistent IF practices may also place greater stress on already weakened hormone functions, including the adrenal and thyroid glands, in women training for a marathon. However, one recent review concluded that if athletes maintain their total intake of calories and micronutrients, and their sleep quality, they would be unlikely to experience any negative performance effects.

The downsides for runners include the timing of the fasting days. If you are running four or five times a week, it can be difficult to ensure that your training days do not coincide with a fasting day. If your fasting day only allows 500 calories, for example, your energy levels and fuelling may not allow for you to expend great deals of energy on running. Running when fasting can impact performance, both on that day and through leaving you fatigued and insufficiently recovered for future training.

For women, there is strong evidence that restricted eating practices, including IF, can place the body under greater stress, causing an increase in cortisol and associated weight gain, specifically around the belly, which can significantly detract from training benefits. In conclusion, IF could work. I know plenty of endurance runners who fast intermittently and consistently run at a good level, but it is imperative to look at the whole picture of your health to see if it really is the right thing for you.

Ultrarunning

"Ultrarunning is just an eating and drinking competition, with a little bit of running thrown in." - Ann Trason

Ultrarunning is a step up from a marathon. Officially, it is any distance beyond the standard marathon of 42km (26.2 miles). The events are often 50km, 100km, 50 miles or even 100 miles. Some ultras can be run within a day, while others are spread over several, and formats vary from laps of a track to hilly trails.

Training for an ultra event requires commitment, dedication and determination, and if you want to be successful, your nutrition requires the same discipline. Running these distances and the recovery that entails demands constant, specific nutrition interventions. The energy needs of endurance runners are hugely increased compared with runners training for shorter distances. You will need to eat larger quantities of food and the requirements for essential vitamins and minerals are also significantly increased to keep you running strong, healthy and injury free. Individual nutrition requirements are, of course, determined by training load, goals, specific individual needs, environment, body composition goals and any underlying health issues.

Nutrition for ultrarunning

When training for and running the ultramarathon distance, the appropriate type, quantity and timing of fuel for your body is vital to ensure you have enough energy to complete your long runs. There is no doubt that ultrarunning is tiring, energy sapping and tough on your body, but ultimately it's extremely rewarding.

There are two main sources of fuel for exercise: carbohydrates and fats. During shorter, faster runs, your body primarily uses carbohydrate (glucose) for energy, but as the distance increases, with speed typically decreasing, there is a shift towards relying more on fat as a primary fuel source. Carbohydrate is still important, but the balance shifts a little and fat becomes more critical for energy production. This reliance on fat for fuel helps to spare carbohydrate stores, of which there is a limited supply. This is beneficial for endurance events, because when you run too low on carbohydrates, fatigue quickly kicks in.

In recent years, there has been plenty of debate over whether a high-carbohydrate or high-fat diet is best for endurance runners, with the general conclusion reached that there are benefits and downsides to both, with the final choice being down to individual preference depending on training, age and genetic tendencies.

One drawback of a high-carbohydrate diet, especially when it's high in refined sugar, is blood sugar imbalances from chronically stimulated insulin levels, which can result in fatigue and weight gain. Although you can reduce your reliance on carbohydrates, it is not possible to eliminate it.

Initially, studies reported that high-fat diets are more likely to improve endurance running when compared with high-carbohydrate ones. However, it was later found that these endurance benefits were only seen at relatively low intensities, such as you might experience on a long training run incorporating several walking sections. Once exercise intensity increased, as would occur during a race, so did carbohydrate requirements, and athletes on a high-fat diet lacked sufficient glycogen to continue for long periods.

Fuelling during ultrarunning

So, what do ultrarunners eat during their training runs and races? The short answer is, anything and everything! The rules seem to change over and above the marathon distance, from a heavy reliance on energy gels to eating real food. In my experience, ultrarunning is all about eating actual food, which perhaps is what appeals to many of us. One great American ultrarunner, Ann Trason, reportedly said, "Ultrarunning is just an eating and drinking competition, with a little bit of running thrown in."

Fundamentally, the food you choose to fuel yourself with during ultra-training and racing needs to be tasty (to you) and palatable, providing carbohydrates a little at a time, with small amounts of protein and fat, as required. Although you may not feel hungry, it is imperative that you do eat regularly, so finding foods that appeal to you is a key part of the prep for these runs.

During my second ultramarathon, I ate loads of salted pretzels, peanut butter sandwiches, watermelon and iced biscuits. At the aid stations, I was like a kid in a sweet shop, grabbing handfuls of pretzels and biscuits. The weather was super hot and my body was craving extra salt. Rice cakes can work well, as do flapjacks and granola bars, bananas, jam sandwiches and jelly sweets. Pouches of baby food are allegedly commonplace during ultra events, though I have yet to try this myself.

Hydration for ultrarunning

As with any distance, it is important to start every training run well hydrated. This requires a consistent, regular intake of caffeine-free fluid throughout each day leading up to training or racing. Drinking a glass of water every few hours, perhaps in between each meal and snack, is a good strategy.

Replacing fluid loss during and after each training run is also vital. Bearing in mind that thirst is a poor indicator of hydration status and fluid needs, it's worth considering your individual sweat loss and environmental factors. Hot or humid weather can lead to greater body fluid loss than when it's cooler, so your hydration needs depend primarily on your environment, while, of course, keeping in mind distance and intensity.

Hydration packs and vests are a vital piece of kit for any budding ultrarunner, because you must carry fluids and other necessities such as your phone, torch, cash, a waterproof and a basic first aid kit yourself. Most hydration packs comfortably carry 1 litre of water, which should see you through a few hours. For female runners, your choice of hydration pack will be personal, depending on your body shape and size. It is imperative to use one that is comfortable, because you'll be wearing it for a long time. Some vests have water bottles positioned in pockets at the front of your chest, which can be troublesome for women with larger breasts, as they sit in the wrong place, causing discomfort. So, be prepared to try a few options.

Recovery nutrition

When training for an ultramarathon, the distances and durations you undertake place huge stress on your body as a whole, so nutritional strategies that help to reduce resulting muscular damage and associated inflammation are necessary. If the terrain you run on includes hills, which many ultrarunners favour, nutrition to support muscle repair becomes even more important.

Protein is crucial for repairing muscles between runs, as it supports muscle strength and power. Studies report that consuming an absolute minimum of 1.6g of protein per kg of body weight per day is necessary, while upper levels vary depending on training and individual needs. As discussed back in Chapter 2, more recent research suggests that consuming more moderate quantities of protein regularly throughout the day is the most efficient way for the body to repair muscles. See page 51 for examples of what 20g of protein looks like.

Focus on iron

Low iron stores are a notoriously common issue for female endurance runners. Iron is essential for creating haemoglobin, the protein in red blood cells responsible for transporting oxygen around the blood. Muscles need oxygen to function properly, and without enough you may feel fatigued and be unable to perform to your aerobic capability.

Female athletes are at a greater risk than male athletes of having low iron stores. This is primarily due to monthly blood loss during menstruation.

Pale skin and brittle nails are two of the most common symptoms of iron-deficiency anaemia, which is the next step along from iron deficiency, but low iron is not always easy to identify. If you are at all feeling below par, it might be worth asking your GP for a blood test to check your ferritin (iron) stores, as even a mild deficiency can impair running performance by reducing your energy levels.

The best way to protect yourself from iron deficiency is through eating a variety of food. There is no getting away from the fact that the body more easily absorbs iron from meat sources, reportedly as much as 35 per cent of the iron in beef, fish and poultry, yet only 2 to 20 per cent of the iron in grains and vegetables, also called non-heme iron. Vegan endurance runners are, therefore, at a greater risk of having low iron stores, though with careful planning and food consideration, this can be avoided. Beans, lentils, dark leafy greens and whole grains, including quinoa, are useful vegan sources of iron.

Immune function in endurance runners

Immune function is especially important when you are training for long periods of time. Endurance exercise such as running has been shown to benefit your immune system, both in the short and long-term, which is partly due to physical activity clearing bacteria out of airways and lungs, which may reduce the likelihood of succumbing to a cold. Intense exercise also promotes antibody activity and increases the production of white blood cells that can fight infection.

However, excessive exercise can suppress the immune system, making ultrarunners more susceptible to cold and flu infections after a long training run. Studies report that exercise-induced immune suppression is typically mild and temporary, yet it can be a cause for concern if training volume and intensity increases too far. The 'J' curve model suggests that moderate exercise improves immune function to a certain point, after which it is depleted and the risk of upper respiratory infection increases, which can interfere with training and recovery. The greater mileage you run, the more rest and nutritional support you need.

Nutritional support for immune function

A healthy diet of whole, natural foods, including 8 to 10 portions of vegetables and fruits a day and a variety of whole grains, nuts, seeds, pulses and beans goes a long way towards supporting a strong immune function.

Additionally, there are specific nutrients that ultrarunners require:

✓ Carotenes – these are powerful antioxidants shown to enhance the integrity of the respiratory tract. They are found in yellow and orange-coloured vegetables, such as carrots, squash, sweet potatoes, red and orange peppers and tomatoes. These are great vegetables to include as part of your daily diet.

✓ Vitamin D – as well as being an important vitamin for strong bones, there is a growing body of evidence supporting vitamin D as essential for a robust immune function. Studies support the avoidance of vitamin D deficiency in female athletes to maintain immunity and prevent upper respiratory illness. Following long, hard bouts of running there is a window of immune suppression where you are more susceptible to viruses. This could be a good time to consider taking a vitamin D supplement, unless you already know that your vitamin D levels are high. Simple finger prick blood tests that you can do at home are available from testing companies such as Thriva and Medichecks.

✓ Vitamin C – this is an especially important micronutrient for endurance runners, as it aids the growth and repair of all body tissues, including tendons, ligaments and blood vessels, in addition to helping the body maintain bone tissue. As vitamin C is unable to be stored in the body, a regular supply needs to be obtained through your diet, and the best way to do this is from regularly consuming colourful fresh vegetables and fruits. Some studies report that high doses of vitamin C can improve recovery after intense and long duration running. A 2013 study on a group of female athletes found that vitamin C supplementation of 250mg per day for four weeks significantly reduced oxidative stress markers, allowing the athletes to recover quickly and continue training.

✓ Zinc – endurance exercise appears to reduce zinc levels in the body for several days, potentially leaving ultramarathon runners more prone to colds and upper respiratory tract infections. High sweat rates are thought to be to blame for zinc depletion, so after training it's important to replenish your levels through eating poultry, red meat, seafood, beans and nuts.

SECTION 3

AFTER CARE

You are onto the final section of the book – the last push before the finish line! Appropriately, this section is all about after care. But perhaps that's misleading, as sleep and trying to remain injury free should be priorities for runners, not an afterthought. Injuries in female runners are all too common, so I wanted to share my knowledge of nutritional interventions that can either aggravate or heal them. As for sleep, we all know how fundamental getting enough kip is to health and strong running. In Chapter 10, I'll share with you exactly what to eat and what to avoid in order to sleep consistently well.

CHAPTER 9

INJURIES AND DOMS

It's a rare runner indeed who has never suffered with aches and pains or some sort of injury. But don't be put off if you are a brand new runner, because once you have read and implemented everything in this chapter, you will be in the perfect place to avoid them.

Sadly, I know a thing or two about injury, having experienced stress fractures and muscular aches at various stages of my running journey. I also have personal experience of how nutrition can impact both injury likelihood and recovery. If you like, I have the nutrition dos and don'ts.

I will state here that even top-notch, personalised functional sports nutrition won't guarantee that you will never experience an injury. You must also factor in sensible training. However, what nutrition does do is reduce the likelihood of an injury and improve the recovery time should you be unfortunate enough to sustain one. What you put into your body can provide the appropriate nutrients to help it heal effectively and quickly.

Whether you are reading this chapter while nursing an injury or thinking ahead to avoiding one, you will learn all the essentials of nutrition necessary for healing and healthy running. Please note: for detailed advice regarding injuries and rehabilitation, contact a registered sports injury professional.

Stress fractures

Stress fractures are very painful and can take a long time to fully heal. In this section, I'll explain exactly what stress fractures are, why female runners commonly suffer with them, and how they are both helped and hindered by nutrition.

Stress fractures are small, fine cracks in the bone, which are generally caused from repeated stress over time, hence the name. In runners, they typically occur in the lower leg and foot bones, where the body bears the most weight.

These types of injuries are not always easy to pinpoint. Common symptoms include pain and sometimes swelling, usually in a specific area of the foot or leg. Although stress fractures are uncomfortable, they tend not to manifest as a constant pain, which can lull you into a false sense of security regarding the extent of the injury and how well it is healing. This is partly why they can take a good while to heal – we simply don't give them enough time to fully recover before we go out running again. Time and rest are crucial.

Reasons for getting stress fractures

Poor biomechanics (the way your whole body moves while running), training errors and a lack of strength training are the most common causes of stress fractures. You don't need to be running a super high mileage to develop a stress fracture. In fact, new runners increasing their distance while training for a big event are more likely to develop them than runners who already regularly run long distances. In terms of biomechanics, runners who overstride, landing mainly on their heels, tend to experience tibial stress fractures in the lower part of their legs. Those runners with a forefoot strike are more likely to suffer stress fractures in their feet, due to the increased load on their ankle and foot bones.

Be conscious of what you wear on your feet, too. Changing your running style or swapping to more minimal footwear too quickly can significantly increase the risk of stress fractures. It's best to make an adjustment gradually, just as you would when training for a longer distance event.

The surface you run on plays a role in the development of both soft tissue and bone injuries. Softer surfaces, such as grass and sand, reduce the impact on your body, so why not invest in some trail shoes and embrace the mud?! Road running may feel easier in wintry weather and quite possibly give you a speed advantage, but weigh those benefits up against the potential injury risks. When I trained for my first road marathon, I ran solely on roads. There were no trails for me back then, and I suffered with niggles and injuries. Yet since swapping to trail running, and taking more recovery time, I haven't experienced a single stress fracture.

Recovery after running is key to staving off injury. Your body may be able to handle higher mileage and poor biomechanics if your nutrition, sleep and stress levels are on top form, but if you have a lot going on, are sleeping badly and making poor food choices then your body could well respond differently.

RED-S

Research shows that female runners tend to suffer with stress fractures more often than male ones. Stress fractures are also more than four times more common in athletes suffering from RED-S, which stands for Relative Energy Deficiency in Sport. RED-S is a term that involves the female athlete triad of decreased bone density, low energy availability and menstrual dysfunction, which can become evident with any combination of stress fracture, low BMI and irregular or absent periods. Younger athletes during the peak time of growth and development can be particularly at risk. However, RED-S can occur at any age. In this section, I cover bone density and low energy availability, including specific nutritional strategies that can help. Refer to Chapter 3 for nutrition for healthy menstrual function.

Bone density

Low bone mineral density (BMD) is a complex issue that occurs more frequently in women over the age of 50, because this is when bone building starts to exceed bone formation. Low bone mass means your bones are getting weaker, and it's a precursor to osteopenia, which itself comes before osteoporosis (also known as brittle bone disease). Osteoporosis occurs when bone density is lost, leaving weak and fragile bones that are more at risk of fracturing and breaking. When it comes to bone health, being forewarned is forearmed, because action can be taken to slow down the progression of bone loss.

Weight-bearing exercise, of which running is obviously one option, is vital for strong bones, though doing it will not preclude you from developing osteoporosis in later life. Too many complexities in the body are at play to make that assumption. Some studies report that vegetarians are at lower risk of developing weak bones. This is partly because plant foods contain the trace mineral boron, which has a positive effect on calcium absorption. It seems that fewer incidences of osteoporosis among vegetarians are due to them losing less bone strength rather than them having stronger bones to begin with.

Nutritional support for decreased bone density

The nutrients to focus on for strong bones include vitamin D, vitamin K, magnesium, calcium, silicon and boron. These act synergistically, meaning they complement each other.

- ✓ Oily fish, dairy products, eggs and mushrooms are useful sources of vitamin D. See page 57 for more on vitamin D and how best to get enough through the food you eat.

- ✓ Vitamin K is found in fermented foods, such as soybeans, sauerkraut and kimchi, as well as in leafy green vegetables like cabbage, kale and broccoli.

- ✓ The mineral silicon, which strengthens connective tissue, is found in unrefined grains and root vegetables. There is some in milk and beer, too, though I am in no way advocating drinking beer as a magical cure for stress fractures! Silicon is also found in good quantities in onions and leafy green vegetables, so there's no reason why vegans can't obtain enough of it from a well-balanced diet.

If you have low BMD

If your BMD is low, there are some things to avoid, as they can make your bones even weaker.

For instance, while an occasional fizzy drink is fine, drinking them regularly over time can increase your risk of stress fractures and slow down your recovery time.

Fizzy soft drinks are strongly associated with osteoporosis because the phosphoric acid they contain leads to lower calcium but higher phosphate levels in the blood. This imbalance encourages your body to pull out calcium from your bones, which obviously reduces bone density.

Try and avoid excess coffee, sugar and alcohol consumption, too. Too much of these can also result in more calcium being leached from your bones, contributing to low bone density.

Low energy availability

Low energy availability can show up as a low BMI, but that's not always the case. Sometimes it appears as low energy.

In its simplest form, low energy availability is not eating enough for the training you are doing. Female runners who have a low energy intake may not be getting adequate vital vitamins and minerals to run, recover and function optimally, putting them at much greater risk of injury.

The difficult question to answer when it comes to body weight is how low is too low? Your BMI is one way to assess your weight, but it has its flaws, as it does not take into account your age, bone mass or muscle mass.

Your ideal body weight is unique to you and very much depends on your life stage. As you get older, it is completely natural to settle at a different and often higher healthy base weight. If you tried to get back to how much you weighed 30 years ago, your body weight could easily become too low for you right now, so please don't do it.

Although your weight is the most obvious way of assessing if energy expenditure (calories burnt) is exceeding energy intake (calories consumed), resulting in weight loss, it does not always provide the whole picture. You want to be thinking about your energy levels, body composition, sleep and mood. These things all indicate whether you are a healthy weight and getting all the nutrients you need. If you feel frail, weak and lacking in energy, no matter what you weigh you could be at greater risk of sustaining a running injury. If you notice you're more irritable than usual, aren't sleeping well and are frequently feeling low or below par then be careful, too, because these are also indicators that you're not getting enough of the necessary nutrients to support your body.

Nutritional support for low energy availability

Start by incorporating more whole foods into your daily diet, with regular meals and snacks.

For those of you who enjoy running longer distances and challenging yourself with races and events, it can sometimes feel difficult to eat enough to sustain your lifestyle. This is where energy-dense foods can be very useful.

These include:

- ✓ Avocados
- ✓ Nuts and seeds
- ✓ Nut butters
- ✓ Meat
- ✓ Oily fish
- ✓ Cheese
- ✓ Eggs

✓ Butter

✓ Olive oil

That is not to say you have free reign over these food choices; moderation is still important for health, but certainly a little bit extra now and then could do you the world of good.

As already discussed in Chapter 2, alcohol depletes B vitamins, iron and zinc, so regularly drinking booze on top of not eating enough for the training you do can compound the problem of not getting enough vital vitamins and minerals. As such, it's advisable to increase your intake of wholegrains and lean protein.

What this all means

Research wholeheartedly supports diet, particularly one low in calcium, magnesium and vitamin D, as playing a role in the occurrence of stress fractures in female runners. By focusing on a diet that is rich in these vitamins and minerals, you can potentially lower the risk of sustaining stress fractures. Sadly, though, the food you eat will not eliminate the risk completely.

I personally see a stress fracture, or any type of pain, as a warning sign. It's a chance to assess your diet and training to avoid the pain getting worse or developing another injury in the future. By making the right changes to the food you eat, and by incorporating more bone-supportive nutrients, you will be helping your body to run stronger for longer.

Soft tissue injuries

Unfortunately, soft tissue injuries, such as knee pain, ITB syndrome, shin splints and plantar fasciitis, are common in runners. Taking the following smart nutritional steps at the first sign of pain or tightness can reduce the chance of developing a full-blown running injury.

I won't delve into specific running injuries, but they do all have something in common that can be addressed through your diet: inflammation.

Soft tissue injuries all feature an element of excess inflammation in specific parts of the body. The key word here is 'excess'. Some inflammation is necessary, as it is part of the healing process, helping you to fight infection and injury, but constant, chronic inflammation destroys rather than heals.

Unfortunately, there isn't much research on nutritional strategies to improve soft tissue function. What there is points to certain amino acids, including proline and lysine, in addition to vitamin C, being able to improve collagen synthesis. Gelatine, a type of beef collagen made from the tendons and ligaments of cows, is rich in proline and lysine. Research shows that some athletes have seen positive responses to injury recovery and collagen production from taking gelatine supplements. However, larger scale clinical trials are needed to verify these results.

Antioxidants genetics

Antioxidants can be helpful in healing soft tissue injuries and strengthening your body to reduce the likelihood of succumbing to an injury in the first place. Here, Dr Eve Pearce gives her take on how our genetic makeup can influence the way our body responds to inflammation.

The genetics of antioxidants and running

Without oxygen, you wouldn't be able to run very far. During sustained training, we use vast amounts of oxygen, up to 15 times more than when we are at rest. As our muscles work harder, we need to breathe in more oxygen to release energy from metabolic fuels, which produces more carbon dioxide to breathe out. However, as it is an unstable molecule, oxygen has a shortcoming. Everyone alive is subject to oxidative stress, where oxygen converts into free radicals (chemicals that can cause damage to body tissues). But because we consume more oxygen while running, we also produce many more free radicals. A low level of free radical production is necessary for regular repeated muscle training and improvement. As we exercise, we cause small damage to muscles, and as we recover, they become that much stronger. But if we exceed a level of free radicals that our body is comfortable with, oxidative stress also partly contributes to muscle fatigue, making it hard to run again the next day. The natural solution to free radicals is antioxidants, which neutralise them and dampen their effects. There are two types of antioxidants: exogenous and endogenous. Exogenous antioxidants come from our diet, mainly fruits and vegetables. Research has shown that antioxidant-rich foods offer recovery benefits to runners and other endurance athletes. Endogenous antioxidants are enzymes produced by the body that act in the same way. The MnSOD gene is responsible for producing manganese. This enzyme is an essential first step in a pathway to removing free radicals, and a genetic variant is associated with a change in its efficiency. This change is quite common and found in around 50 per cent of Caucasians. A study looking at this genetic variation in regular runners has identified an association with exercise recovery. Carriers have increased activity of this cellular antioxidant enzyme, which sounds like a good thing. However, research suggests that this leads to the increased clearance of free radicals when the body is subjected to oxidative stressors such as running. As a result of this initial free radical-removing step, and the resulting increased activity, there is a build-up of a secondary by-product known as peroxide. This causes damage to the body. While it's usually cleared by antioxidants from our diet in a secondary reaction, if there isn't a plentiful supply to keep up with its production, there may be increased oxidative stress and low-grade inflammation. So, it's important for those carrying this variation to consume an antioxidant-rich diet.

Injuries and the menstrual cycle

Interestingly, it seems there is a higher incidence of both soft tissue and musculoskeletal injuries when women undertake intense physical activity during the first part of their menstrual cycle, the follicular phase, and around ovulation. During this time, oestrogen levels are elevated, and it is thought that this hormonal change contributes somehow to the tendons being more elastic, making injuries more likely. However, the same studies also report that intense running during the follicular phase has a protective effect against DOMS. So, there's good news and there's bad. Either way, studies have been small, and the research is currently inconclusive.

Nutritional strategies for inflammation

If you do succumb to a soft tissue injury, then an anti-inflammatory diet could help to heal your body faster. The foods to focus on are primarily the basics of a healthy, balanced diet. These include:

✓ A variety of colourful fruits and vegetables

✓ Lean protein, including beans and pulses

✓ Omega-3 foods, such as oily fish and flaxseed

✓ Wholegrain carbohydrates

✓ Nuts and seeds

✓ Beans and pulses

✓ Extra virgin olive oil

✓ Herbs and spices, such as ginger, turmeric and garlic

When recovering from a soft tissue injury, you also really want to be cutting out, or at least minimising, foods that can increase inflammation in your body, also called pro-inflammatory foods.

These include:

» Added sugars like table sugar
» High-fructose corn syrup, partially hydrogenated oils, found in processed foods
» Pasta and bread made from refined white carbohydrates
» Artificial trans-fats found in packaged foods
» Excess saturated fats from fatty processed meats, such as sausages, hot dogs, ham and salami

Coffee

Some studies have suggested that drinking coffee may delay injury recovery.

Although coffee does have many general health benefits, including moderate coffee consumption potentially lowering the risk of cardiovascular disease and Alzheimer's in some women compared with non-coffee drinkers, most research points to it delaying healing due to the way it constricts blood vessels and reduces blood flow. In order to heal, injuries require more blood flow, not less.

Of course, caffeine can affect people differently, so you don't necessarily need to cut it out when you are suffering with an injury, but you might well benefit from having a think about how much you currently drink and then moderating your consumption for a time. Personally, when I have an injury niggle, I do tend to cut right back on coffee and moderate the less healthy parts of my diet, such as convenience snacks – including bread sticks and crisps – and alcohol.

Injuries and mood

When it comes to injury and nutrition, I feel that it's not about depriving yourself of the nice things in life, but rather getting your mindset geared towards eating the best possible diet, so that you can get back to your beloved running sooner. That thought makes me happy and always gets me through my cravings and difficult days.

Also bear in mind that if you currently have an injury and aren't able to get out running then your mood may be lower than usual. As well as the pain or discomfort you may be feeling, the mere fact you are unable to exercise in the way you want can make you feel rubbish. I know it can be difficult in practice, but this is precisely the time to take the greatest possible care of yourself through nutritious food.

What this all means

Foods that are good for women to eat when dealing with injury and low mood are ones that are colourful, nutritious and uplifting. The anti-inflammatory foods I have already mentioned tick all those boxes.

✓ Turmeric, for example, in a curry or a warm, milky drink, is anti-inflammatory and a beautifully uplifting golden colour.

✓ Beetroot and vibrant orange peppers always make their way into my shopping basket, along with fish and fresh herbs.

Although there is limited research around how food looks in relation to mental health and injury healing, what has been done is overwhelmingly positive. Colourful salads and flashes of colour in an otherwise plain-looking dish have been shown to have a feel-good factor that improves the enjoyment of eating and reduces anxiety and depression. These are the foods to focus on when you are healing and in need of comfort, encouragement and inspiration.

DOMS

DOMS (Delayed-onset muscle soreness) is muscle pain that strikes 24-72 hours after exercise. DOMS occurs most commonly in response to high-intensity or long duration exercise, or after doing something different from usual. Marathon runners famously tend to suffer in the few days after a race. There are plenty of stories of people sitting down after their big run and not being able to get back up again. When DOMS hits, stairs can pose a particular problem post-marathon. My top tip is to walk downstairs backwards, and never in high heels. The day after my first marathon, I became famous in the office not for my athletic achievement but for the fact I removed my shoes every single time I had to navigate the stairs, which was a lot!

While working on this chapter, I was interested to know who suffers from DOMS more, women or men. Research shows that men may report greater and more frequent delayed-onset muscle pain than their female counterparts. This is possibly due to women having greater levels of oestrogen, resulting in less creatine kinase, an enzyme found in the heart muscle, brain tissue and skeletal muscle that results in fewer incidents of muscle soreness. Men tend to have lower oestrogen and greater creatine kinase in their blood, indicating greater muscle damage. It seems that female hormones may play a role in muscle soreness and recovery time, this time in our favour. But do not celebrate yet. You may be able to run further than your husband or brother before the soreness kicks in, but you can still suffer. And sore, stiff muscles hurt a lot.

If your legs aren't used to it, downhill running can often result in DOMS. This is because it's a source of eccentric stress, a type of movement that lengthens a muscle at the same time as it is being contracted. Studies on the effect of DOMS on the legs show that it results in swelling, muscular tension, loss of coordination and a reduced range of motion.

Nutritional interventions for DOMS

There are two ways of approaching nutritional support, either preventative or therapeutic. Here, I'll cover both the foods you can eat to reduce the likelihood of experiencing muscle soreness and those that will help you to recover more quickly.

Montmorency tart cherries

This delicious fruit has been well studied in relation to its effect on muscle soreness. The variety of sour cherry, which is grown in Europe, Canada and the US, is extremely high in numerous plant compounds that provide antioxidant and anti-inflammatory properties. Drinking

30ml of concentrate Montmorency tart cherry juice, either neat or diluted, twice a day can accelerate recovery from muscle-induced damage. This is equivalent to eating around sixty cherries, so this is one instance where a supplement product is by far the most practical and convenient option. There is evidence to show that Montmorency cherries also contain melatonin, a hormone that regulates the sleep-wake cycle; therefore, it can also improve sleep quality. Drinking 30ml of concentrate around one hour before bed may be an effective way to improve sleep and ease muscle damage in one fell swoop, leaving you ready to take on your next training session with energy and enthusiasm.

Ginger and turmeric

Spices, including ginger and turmeric, are rich in antioxidants and highly anti-inflammatory. They help to exert a therapeutic effect on sore muscles by blocking inflammatory chemicals and enzymes. Antioxidants are vital for helping to 'mop up' damaging free-radical molecules that are produced during intense exercise. Plus, they are great for your immune function. Unfortunately, research suggests that using spices extensively in your cooking is not enough to prevent DOMS. Muscle soreness mainly occurs in response to the type of running and exercise you do, rather than from what you eat, although some foods, such as sugar, are known to make the effects of inflammation worse.

Turmeric is a bright yellow powder that is often used in cooking to flavour curries. It is understood to help relieve pain, stiffness and inflammation due to its active chemical curcumin, which may make DOMS less severe and speed up recovery times. If you can get hold of fresh turmeric, a knobbly looking root with a gorgeous, orange-coloured flesh, then great. Alternatively, good quality powdered turmeric is easy to come by. I always have a jar stashed away in my kitchen cupboard.

Turmeric tea recipe:

This is a super-warming, anti-inflammatory healing tea, which is perfect for drinking after wintry day runs.

» 1 tsp turmeric powder
» 1 tsp honey
» ½ lemon
» Black pepper

Method:

In a small bowl, mix the turmeric powder and honey into a smooth paste.

Add a squeeze of lemon juice and a few grinds of black pepper to bring out the flavour and aid the absorption of the turmeric.

Add a little hot water, mix thoroughly and drink. Down in one is my preference!

Ginger is another great spice for calming down sore muscles after running, as it has similar anti-inflammatory properties to turmeric. Supplements can help, as can consuming fresh or powdered ginger. A therapeutic dose of fresh ginger is around 2g per day, which is equivalent to about 1.5 teaspoons. Ginger and lemon combine well in a tea, and it's great to drink after running, as it will help to moderate the effects of inflammation and boost immune function. Another option is to massage ginger oil into sore areas. Ginger-based oils and balms are fabulous for warming up specific muscles and getting more blood flow to the area, which itself promotes healing. You may find that a combination of methods works best for you. Ginger is also fabulous for your digestion, effectively calming nausea and soothing an irritable gut.

Caffeine

One study on caffeine found that 5mg per kg of body weight consumed 24 hours prior to and 48 hours after resistance training resulted in a significant reduction in the incidence of DOMS compared with the placebo group. One reason for this is thought to be the blocking effect of caffeine on adenosine receptors, which may reduce DOMS by deactivating the central nervous system. Simply put, caffeine may be capable of blunting pain and inflammation.

To reap the benefit of caffeine, you need to consume enough. Research shows that lower dosages have little if any effect on delayed-onset muscle soreness. Putting quantities into context, 5mg of caffeine per kg of body weight is equivalent to 350mg of caffeine per day for a 70kg (11 stone) runner; that's about two cups of coffee. For some of you, that may be a typical daily intake, in which case the effects on muscle soreness may be less pronounced. This is because habitual coffee consumption can cause your body to build up a tolerance to caffeine, meaning its pain-relieving effects may not be as apparent. Therefore, to receive the benefit, you would need to drink more than your body is used to. For others, two cups of coffee may not be an option if it impacts sleep or anxiety too much. No matter what the research says, always consider what is the right thing for you.

Taurine

Taurine is an organic acid that is primarily found in skeletal muscle. It has been shown to work against cytokines, which are chemicals that can cause damage and inflammation to our cells. Therefore, taurine may play a role in preventing the root cause of DOMS. Studies on taurine supplementation in reducing muscular pain have been positive. The most effective dose seems to be 2g taken 3 times a day.

One question that often comes up in my nutrition clinic concerns whether we can consume enough taurine through our food, without taking supplements. Currently, there is no official recommended daily intake for taurine, however, studies indicate that on average, most women consume around 400mg through their food per day, which is enough for general health. Cheese, pork, eggs and the dark meat of chicken and turkey are useful sources of taurine. As you can see from the table below, it is generally found in greater concentrations in animal products, so if you follow a vegan diet you might want to consider supplementation, though bear in mind that our bodies do produce some taurine naturally.

Food sources of taurine:	Amounts in mg:
1 medium egg	350mg
40g of hard cheese	500mg
85g of pork	550mg

What this all means

There are practical steps that you can take to reduce the likelihood of experiencing DOMS, such as gradually increasing your training intensity and duration.

By eating a diet rich in anti-inflammatory foods, such as colourful fruits and vegetables and herbs and spices, and by ensuring you consume sufficient protective nutrients like taurine, you will be giving your body the best chance of preventing muscle soreness after exercise.

If you do experience DOMS, then you now know some of the best foods to effectively reduce soreness, helping you to quickly return to an exercise or training programme.

CHAPTER 10

SLEEP

You might be wondering why there is a whole chapter dedicated to sleep in a book about nutrition and running for women. The answer is because rest, of which sleep is a major part, is vital to your health and running performance. You could last for several hours without water and a few days without food (if absolutely necessary), but even one night of no sleep impacts your ability to think clearly and recover from training. Therefore, it makes perfect sense to see sleep as a tool for enhancing athletic performance.

Why do female runners need sufficient sleep?

You need enough sleep for both your body and mind to recharge. Sleep also helps your body remain healthy and fight off illness, as well as repairing muscles and cells after exercise. Sleep also enhances running performance, both physically and mentally.

Women tend to report more common and severe sleep problems than men, which is thought to be partly down to hormonal fluctuations. What these scientific studies don't discuss is how much lifestyle factors influence sleep quality and quantity. As I talked about in Chapter 5, a female runner's life load can, at certain times, be overwhelming, which more than likely impacts sleep. For example, although a runner with a baby or toddler may need more sleep than ever to recover from training sessions and early morning wake-up calls from little people, their likelihood of getting enough sleep is slim. We can cope for a while on sleep deprivation, but there does come a tipping point, where health and running performance are negatively impacted due to a lack of rest and recovery.

Immune function

Without sufficient sleep, your body's immune function is compromised. Even though running, and in fact any form of exercise, has been proven to strengthen the immune system, you will not reap all of the benefits without getting plenty of sleep and rest. When you are sleep deprived, your immune function must work harder, leaving you more susceptible to infections and illness. Feeling tired and rundown is usually your body telling you something – specifically that you need to rest and sleep more. See page 158 for more on immunity function in female endurance runners and the nutritional strategies that can help support a strong, healthy immune system.

Mental and physical performance

Sleep allows our body and mind to relax and recover. When we don't get enough, we can't perform at our best. The impact of poor sleep on how well you think and function should not be ignored, yet sadly, it's often put at the bottom of the list. Mental function after a poor night's rest is reduced, leaving you uncoordinated, with slower reaction times. This puts you at risk of tripping over on your run.

You may have noticed that when you are sleep deprived, you are less able to produce a quick turn of speed and feel less sure-footed. I can certainly feel the difference after a bad night's sleep, as what is usually an enjoyable run feels like an unpleasant slog. Of course, running outside in the fresh air also has the ability to do wonders for boosting mental fatigue and getting you through the rest of the day. Sometimes, a dose of fresh air and exercise is just what your body needs to have a great day, regardless of how tired you initially feel.

Injuries

It's undeniable that a chronic lack of sleep can put runners at greater risk of injury, because without sufficient overnight rest, muscle growth and recovery, immune system function and inflammatory response are altered.

If you are currently dealing with a running injury, sufficient sleep is vital for a speedy recovery, which is partly because the growth hormones that enhance injury repair are secreted during deep sleep. At regular points in the sleep cycle, healing chemicals and hormones are released, which reduce inflammation and give the body the right conditions to repair and heal. While it is true that chronic pain from an injury can make getting deep, restful sleep trickier, a good night's slumber undoubtedly improves chronic pain and inflammation, giving the body a greater chance of healing.

Factors influencing sleep

Runners who train later in the day may benefit from monitoring and adjusting when they head out, as intense running after around 4pm can cause sleep disruption. This is partly due to adrenaline and cortisol spiking at a time when the body expects and needs these hormone levels to drop. Many of my club runners tell me that they find it difficult to sleep after our Tuesday evening track session, because that feeling of being physically tired yet also wired can be annoyingly persistent. It should be said that not all runners have this problem. Late evening running may work well for you, but it's something to watch out for.

Here, Dr Eve Pearce gives the evidence for how genetics affects sleep and running.

The genetics of sleep and running

The daily rotation of our planet around the sun influences our environment. It gives us predictable seasonal patterns, such as weather and daylight. To adjust to this and aid survival, all organisms have evolved internal controls known as the circadian rhythm, which functions to coordinate physiological responses during the daily 24-hour cycle. This includes sleep-wake cycles and physiological changes, such as to our blood pressure, body temperature and metabolism. These daily rhythms are generated by the coordinated gene expression of our so-called 'internal body clock'. Most of us would agree that we tend to know what time of the day suits us best for doing a workout routine. Genetics can also give us some clues about the functioning of our internal body clock.

CLOCK

A conveniently named gene, CLOCK, encodes a protein that is a vital part of generating circadian rhythms. A SNP (single nucleotide polymorphism) in this gene was found in humans as early as 1998. Those who have this genetic variation were shown to have a preference for evenings, an association which has been replicated many times. Thus, this SNP is associated with your morning or evening preference, i.e., whether you are an early lark or a night owl. Those who prefer the evenings tend to sleep for a shorter time and feel sleepy during the day. This results in less physical activity due to fatigue and a tendency to start daily activities later in the morning. Understanding this genetic predisposition can help with monitoring and adjusting sleep timing for the benefit of your running.

The impact of food and drink on sleep

Caffeine, alcohol, sugar and food intolerances can all negatively impact sleep. Also, even mild dehydration can impede it, and this is a common concern for runners.

Caffeine, the active ingredient in coffee, tea, chocolate and products made with these foods, is a well-known stimulant and sleep disrupter. As Dr Eve Pearce explained on page 134, individuals are either 'fast' or 'slow' metabolisers of caffeine. 'Slow' metabolisers will find that even an 11am coffee can disrupt their sleep, while 'fast' metabolisers may be able to stretch their caffeine curfew until the afternoon.

Alcohol, as already discussed in Chapter 2, is known to affect sleep patterns and REM sleep. I strongly advise against drinking alcohol after a late evening run, as the double impact of heightened stress hormones and elevated blood alcohol levels can severely impact deep restorative sleep.

Consuming an excess of sugar is not only detrimental to your health and running performance, but it can also cause sleep problems. According to a 2016 study, people who regularly consume high-sugar foods tend to sleep less deeply and experience more restlessness at night. Insomnia, a disorder whereby people have difficulty falling or staying asleep, is directly linked to blood sugar imbalances. Having high or low blood sugar at bedtime can make it difficult to achieve restful sleep. Studies report women suffering with insomnia more frequently than men, although men are much more vulnerable to the effects of sleep deprivation. It seems that even though we may not sleep as well as our male counterparts, we can handle it better!

How much sleep do we need?

Sleep requirements vary widely and partly depend on your age and activity level, amongst other things. The well-cited rule of 8 hours of sleep a night is just a convenient guide rather than a strict rule. Because we are all different, some of you will need much more than 8 hours a night, while others will function perfectly well on much less. Now that scientists have delved deeper into how we sleep, it is known that the body goes through 90-minute cycles. Therefore, in order to fit in with these cycles, there is a strong body of evidence building up for people to aim for either 6, 7.5 or 9 hours of sleep a night. The physical stress and exertion of running may mean that you need more rest and sleep than less active individuals.

Nutrition to aid sleep

Along with cutting out or reducing stimulants such as caffeine, alcohol, specific food sensitivities and sugar, there are nutrients and foods that have been shown to improve sleep in some people.

✓ Kiwi fruit – one study found that after four weeks of eating two kiwis an hour before bedtime, sleep was significantly improved, particularly getting to sleep more quickly and sleeping more soundly. Further investigation into the sleep-promoting properties of kiwi fruit is needed, but the initial thinking is that the abundance of antioxidants, folate and serotonin contained in this gorgeous fruit may play a role.

✓ Almonds – these nuts are rich in magnesium and calcium, which are known to promote relaxation and sleep, as well as containing good levels of melatonin and zinc. Research indicates that the powerful combination of melatonin, magnesium and zinc has the ability to help older adults with insomnia to sleep better. There have been few studies done specifically with almonds in relation to sleep, but one found that eating ten almonds a day for two weeks significantly improved sleep quality in a group of students.

✓ Warm milk – there isn't actually any solid research on drinking warm milk in the evening to help with sleep, but its nutritional properties do make it a good candidate. Milk contains tryptophan, an amino acid that can help the body produce the neurotransmitter serotonin, which in turn can induce more restful and deeper sleep, by creating melatonin. Like almonds, milk is also rich in calcium, which is known to promote relaxation. Warm milk can be an especially good choice for runners due to its combination of protein, carbohydrate, calcium and vitamin D, the latter two being useful to support bone health.

✓ Magnesium supplements – a powerhouse of a nutrient, many studies have shown magnesium to play an important role in calming your nervous system and relieving anxiety and depression, which can both interfere with sleep. Although there are many foods that are naturally rich in magnesium, including almonds, cashew nuts, spinach and bananas, eating enough to make a significant difference to sleep can be challenging. For this reason, magnesium supplements, oil sprays and old-fashioned Epsom salt baths can be useful in promoting a deep, restful night's sleep. Epsom salts, so called because they were originally discovered in the town of Epsom in Surrey, are an easily absorbed form of magnesium. 100mg of magnesium glycinate taken one hour before bedtime has been shown to promote deep sleep. Because magnesium is also known to improve muscle recovery, a targeted magnesium oil spray rubbed into your legs before bedtime can be especially useful for runners. Alternatively, relaxing in an Epsom salt bath can work wonders for both the mind and body, particularly after a race or intense training.

Sleep is one of the most enjoyable tools for athletic performance, having the ability to improve both your speed and your recovery. There are plenty of nutritional interventions to try, plus some to avoid, and with a little trial and error, I have no doubt that you will hit upon the right combination for you.

CHAPTER 11

HOW TO CREATE LASTING CHANGE

This chapter has kindly been written by Clare Flaxen, a Cognitive Behavioural Therapist.

How many times have you set yourself goals or made resolutions to form new habits? You may have come up with an intention, something like, "Starting next week, I'm going to exercise every day", or set targets, maybe around changing your diet or upping your training schedule. What tends to happen?

A study by the University of Scranton in the US followed 200 people and their New Year's resolutions. They wanted to see how successful people are with self-motivated change. After a week, 77 per cent of them had kept on track with their intentions (pretty good, but that also means that 23 per cent of them never even really got started). After a month, this dropped to 64 per cent. Six months in, only 46 per cent of the participants were still keeping their resolutions, and when the researchers followed up after two years, only 19 per cent had sustained those changes. Read another way, 81 per cent hadn't managed to keep up with their resolutions long-term. That's a lot of people not managing to make the grade. So, what makes the difference between those who succeed and those who don't? Well, think about this. As you've been reading through this book, you've been picking up information and increasing your knowledge thanks to Helen's expertise. You're clear on your goals and what you need to do to get there. You've made your plan.

Having a clear plan with tangible outcomes and clearly thought-out steps to get there already puts you ahead of the game when it comes to reaching goals.

"A goal without a plan is just a wish." – Antoine de Saint-Exupéry

TIP: if you haven't done this yet, go back and get super specific on your goals and your plan. It's a big deciding factor in those who succeed in moving forward with their goals.

But even with a clear plan in place, how do you make sure you don't fall into that 81 per cent who fail to make their changes stick, and to reach or sustain their ultimate goals?

Let's start on a positive: the fact that you're reading this book and are making a plan already increases your odds of being successful. And for the remainder of this chapter, I'm going to look at two further main areas: understanding how your brain is designed in relation to change and building a strong mindset. I'll show you how to work around the natural tendencies of your brain to create blocks to change and focus on your mindset, which is the key foundation to any change or growth within yourself.

I'm a cognitive behavioural therapist and I know how tricky it can be to change old ways and bring in the new habits needed to reach the goals you've set yourself. I work with people every day on changing the patterns of thinking and behaving that aren't serving them well and are holding them back or creating blocks in their life. I help them work through the cycle of change to create new habits and new ways of seeing themselves in relation to the goals they want to achieve.

I like to think of my job as being a disruptor. I'm:

→ Disrupting the automatic responses that keep you stuck in old ways of doing.

→ Disrupting outdated or inaccurate beliefs about yourself.

→ Disrupting patterns of thinking and the stories you create that hold you back.

And then I'm being a creator:

→ Rewiring your brain with new habits.

→ Creating new ways of seeing yourself, with increased confidence and belief in what's possible to achieve.

→ Adopting a new style of self-talk that keeps you going when doubt, fear or self-sabotage kick in.

As well as working with other people on the changes they want to bring into their lives, I've done this in my life, too. I've made long-term changes to my habits around alcohol, I've become a cold-water swimmer and swum consistently in temperatures I never thought would be possible (let alone enjoyable), and I'm a runner, too, and training for my first half marathon. I know what it's like to try and create long lasting change and to strive to achieve goals that you're sometimes not sure are possible.

In this chapter, we're going to focus on the key areas I use in my work to help people just like you reach their goals and get the benefit and satisfaction of creating long-lasting change.

These are:

→ Understanding the nature of being human and how to work around the design flaws we all have that hold us back from change.

→ Using the psychology of change to help keep you motivated and on track.

→ The all-important mindset piece of the puzzle.

→ Creating habits that become your default setting and part of your identity.

→ Using tools and strategies to make it as easy as possible, and to help it stick.

Ready to get started? Grab yourself a pen and paper, go to: www.helenmortonnutrition.com/resources/how-to-create-lasting-change and download blank PDF sheets to fill in, or open up the Notes app on your phone. You're going to be working through the ideas and strategies in this chapter to make it relevant for you and your goals, and to really make it land.

LEARNING-ACTION-CHANGE

In order for it to become a tangible change, learning needs to be activated. In the same way you can't just read about nutrition or exercise and expect your health or fitness to improve, you need to do more than just understand your mindset and how you're wired – you need to test out what you've learned in life and put the strategies into action.

It's true that you can't change what you don't know. But once you know it, you need to take action. Let's start off by taking a look at how your brain is wired, and why it's *so* resistant to change.

Your brain & change

Your brain *really* doesn't like change. It's hardwired to resist it, and so it has a tendency to sabotage your attempts at bringing in new habits or switching up the way you think about something.

Your brain has two main functions that aren't compatible with change: it wants to be able to predict what happens and it wants to know you're going to be safe. It can be useful to think of your brain as a protective parent or a risk-averse analyst.

Your brain thrives on familiarity. There's safety and predictability in this. It can assess what's likely to happen, formulate patterns and, therefore, a plan. It can let you tick along on autopilot, which is much more straightforward than having to weigh up each action you want to take.

On the other hand, change, or something unfamiliar, takes more energy and brain power. It's uncertain and unclear how things are going to play out. Is it safe? Can you do it? What's going to happen? Your brain wants answers to all of these things!

This is important to know about, because the next time your alarm goes off and instead of going out for that run you hit the snooze button, you will see it as part of the nature of your brain, instead of you just giving up and telling yourself it's not possible for someone like you to make the changes you want. This takes away a layer of blame and self-doubt. Instead of thinking, "See, I can't do this", you can turn it into, "How can I work with my brain and send the message that it's OK and I want to do this?"

There's a big design flaw in the brain's safety mechanisms. Your brain is VERY risk averse and doesn't always stop to differentiate between harmful and helpful change. But what if the change you want is actually a positive one? Something that will be beneficial for you instead of harmful – like exercising more or eating more healthily? And what if your goal is something you're not 100 per cent sure you can achieve, such as running a marathon, but are prepared to train and try for anyway? Your brain confuses the actual risk of physical threat with subjective, perceived risks – pushing your limits in a measured way, for instance, or taking a risk that's not in reality dangerous but might leave you feeling embarrassed or that you might fail at.

As a race, we humans are prepared to take a level of risk in our lives in order to grow, progress and challenge ourselves. But in doing so, we're working against the hardwired nature of our brain. To get around that, you need to bring some conscious awareness to what's at play.

Rewiring the brain

Once you bring conscious awareness to the risk-averse, pattern-loving nature of your brain, you can start to work with it to help bypass its naturally cautious nature. You can start to create new patterns that are in line with your new goals. After all, you know your goals aren't a threat your brain needs to save you from, right?

Working with your brain's neuroplasticity, or its ability to lay down new pathways from new experiences, messages and behaviours to create familiarity, you can formulate habits that become second nature and your default mode of being.

The key things you need to know

If you want to reach your goals, you need to be *specific* in telling your brain what you want it to do. It needs clear instructions and to know what the boundaries are. "I'm going to start running" is too vague. Your brain doesn't know what to do with that and so it shunts you into thinking, "OK, we'll go for a run tomorrow" or, "We'll think about running while we lie on the sofa watching TV and eating biscuits."

So, *get clear* on what your goal is and make it tangible. The more specific, the better. Clear steps make it easier to action and easier for you to give your brain the signals that it's OK to go for it.

Visualise yourself doing it. Once you've got the steps figured out, play it over in your mind. You can help that process of neuroplasticity along by playing mini movies in your mind of you taking the action and doing the things that will get you to your goal.

Help your brain to lay this visualisation down as a *positive memory* by utilising as many senses as possible. For instance, smile while you picture yourself out running, and trigger the all-important reward and pleasure parts of your brain that drive so many of your behaviours. Imagine yourself out running, feeling strong and light. Fill the image with colour, whichever one comes naturally to you as you play the image out in your mind. Set it to music, and as you picture the scene, imagine hearing your favourite running song.

The stronger the image you can create, the stronger your brain will latch onto it and store it away as a time when you had a great experience of moving towards your goal.

» Focus on the journey, not just the end result

A big element that trips people up as they try to reach goals and create new habits is focusing solely on the end result and missing out the steps they'll need to take and the ups and downs that will invariably come.

By all means, visualise the end goal and picture yourself achieving it: your brain needs to see that it's possible. But focus too on the different stages you'll need to go through in order to get there. Acknowledge and accept that it will get messy at times, that things may not go to plan and that you're likely to fall back into old ways at certain points. See it as part of the process, as that way it'll be much easier to pick things up and keep going. Instead of feeling you've failed and giving up, you'll understand that it's part of the journey and that it happens to everyone.

So, picture it being hard some days. Picture yourself having a run that feels heavy and difficult. Picture yourself throwing the healthy eating plan out of the window. But don't end the thought process there. See it through and picture yourself dealing with it. Visualise yourself coping with the runs that feel tough, instead of taking it as evidence that you're not cut out for this. Picture yourself feeling like giving up but keeping going instead. Show yourself that small steps, consistently taken, will lead to big changes.

Instead of letting your inner critic take over when things slip, practise viewing this in a more accepting light and know that the key thing is to keep going.

The path doesn't have to be straight. What's important is that you keep moving along it.

» Know your Big Why

Your motivation is going to wane. It's human nature. The rocket fuel that gets behind you when you first feel inspired to make changes is hard to sustain. Part of creating new, familiar habits is that things can get a bit boring along the way or feel too difficult. Contemplating your Big Why will help you to reconnect with what's important to you.

A big mistake people often make is choosing the wrong WHY

EAT WELL, RUN STRONG – HELEN MORTON

If your why is based on what other people are doing or things you think you should be doing, as opposed to what you really want to do, then you're going to grind to a halt pretty quickly.

Likewise, if it's based on something too surface level, like your weight on the scales or a notion of getting fit, then it's going to be hard to connect to why that really matters to you and how your life will benefit. This is also true of a specific goal like entering a sports competition or pushing yourself in a race – unless you connect with the deeper why on a personal level, it's going to be hard to keep motivated.

Have a think about your Big Why now. What drives you? Why is it important to you? What will it mean to you when you achieve it? How will it benefit your life or the people who matter to you? What will it add to your life? What's the purpose of all this? Get your why solid and your motivation will be far easier to tap into when you need it. Then when you hit a wall or the going gets tough, *why* you're striving to reach your goals will be important in getting you back on track and digging deep into the reserves of your self-discipline and motivation.

When I started cold-water swimming, I was initially just curious to see if I could do it. I had this arbitrary notion in my head that the people I saw heading to the lido near where I live, in the depths of winter, were somehow made of different stuff than me. I wanted to see if I could do it, too. My surface level 'why' was to see how far through winter I could swim, and to get some of the good mental and physical benefits I'd read about. My deeper 'why' was connected to my own sense of self-belief. I wanted to expand my notion of what was possible for me to achieve. If I could swim in freezing temperatures and master my mindset in that situation, I could do the same in the other areas of my life where doubts or fears were holding me back.

Your Big Why will be a strong ally when the going gets tough and you want to quit. So, give it some thought at the start of your journey.

» Remove as many barriers as you can

Your brain will already be resisting change, so you've got to make it as easy as possible for yourself. For instance, if you're ready to start changing your nutrition, remove as many barriers to this as you can.

→ Figure out your What, Where, When and How, and make it as straightforward as possible.

→ What are you going to do? Where will you do it? When will you do it? How will you make it happen?

» Tap into the reward centre of your brain

Your brain has a strong reward driver. We get hooked on cycles of reward and pleasure because this is a much stronger motivator than doing what we know is best for us. This is why we make poor choices so easily and reach for sugar-laden foods instead of healthy snacks, or turn on the TV instead of going out for a run.

The trick is to flip it: focus on what you gain rather than what you lose and make the new behaviour the reward. Make the focus how you feel after your run, when all those wonderful feel-good chemicals are being released. Or think about the freedom you get from being out and moving. Make the healthy option the reward because of the energy you get from it and the reward of making a beneficial choice for the future you.

If you're introducing new habits that you find difficult to get pleasure out of, or you want a helping hand kickstarting them and making them familiar, try using these two techniques:

1. **Piggybacking** – piggyback the new habit onto something you already find enjoyable, such as listening to music you love when you run or making it your podcast time. Make that the reward.

1. **Bootstrap it** – tack it onto something you already do routinely, such as taking your nutritional supplements at the same time as your morning cuppa or straight after you brush your teeth. Take something that you already habitually do and add the new behaviour onto this.

» Make it familiar

The key thing about creating new habits and rewiring your brain is to make the new behaviour so familiar that it becomes second nature and just what you do. You can do this by consistent repetition. Doing the new thing over and over will mean your brain gets used to it and it will become familiar, safe and predictable. And we already know that your brain likes this.

While you're making new habits *familiar*, you'll be making the current patterns you want to change *unfamiliar*. You'll be creating distance between what you used to do and making it seem unfamiliar and separate from you. Switching over the habits will help you to make them stick long-term.

» Make it part of your identity

When you make something familiar and the new norm, you also want to make it part of your identity: something that you do, which is your thing.

"I'm Clare and I'm a runner. I'm Clare and I'm a cold-water swimmer."

It's got way more impact when you see it as a part of you.

» I choose this

When you're laying down your new habits and your natural tendency to revert back to your old ways kicks in, practise the above and add in talking back to your brain. Let it know that you're choosing to do this. Let it know that it's OK, that it doesn't need to protect you right now and that you've got this. Even if it's going to be hard or you're not sure of the outcome, you're still choosing to do it.

Your brain's protective mechanisms can show up in all sorts of ways: avoidance, procrastination, self-sabotage, fear, self-doubt and negative self-talk, to name a few. We're going to look at the mindset part next, and how to tackle the times when your inner critic pipes up, or a fear of failure or judgement from yourself or others holds you back and takes you off course.

But first, take a look at these statements and let's start making a plan for how you'll override or soothe that risk-averse brain of yours:

- → My exercise goal is:
- → My super clear goal is:
- → My Big Why is:
- → What motivates me is:
- → The reward is:
- → I'll make it fun by:
- → I'll make it easy by:
- → I'll make it familiar by:
- → What I'll say to my brain: IT'S OK, I CHOOSE THIS.

Go to www.helenmortonnutrition.com/resources/how-to-create-lasting-change/ to get PDF pages (The Plan, part 1) that you can fill in.

The stages of change – where are you?

A quick, useful exercise is to look at where you're at in the process of change. It'll help you figure out the next steps to take.

Are you:

1. **Thinking about it?**

   There are some changes you've been thinking about making and you're contemplating what life could be like if you made them. Maybe you've started thinking about a goal you'd like to set yourself.

2. Ready to go for it?

   You're feeling motivated! You've set your goals and you're raring to get started. You just need to take that first step.

3. Doing it?

   You've set your targets, and you know what steps you need to take and have started putting them into action.

4. In your groove with it?

   You're in your flow. You've been putting the steps and actions into practise and you're seeing the results. Now the challenge is to keep going with your new habits and make the changes a regular part of your life.

5. Doing it, but have fallen back into old habits?

   Things were going great, but it's tapered off, or out of nowhere you've let everything drop and you're back to your old ways.

Where would you place yourself in this list?

For *all* of these stages, your mindset is going to be key to either getting started or keeping going. Remember, to fall off the wagon is a normal part of the process. Rather than seeing it as a sign of failure or a reason to give up, accept it as something that happens to the best of us and pick things up again. The quicker you can get going and stop wasting energy on feeling bad that you fell back into old ways, the easier it will be to start seeing that motivation-boosting progress again.

You'll also be changing up the inner self-talk that holds you back by saying you're not good enough or can't do this. We'll get to this more in the mindset section, but it's important to start seeing how your actions and thoughts define what you believe about yourself and how you feel. This is an integral part of motivation and continuing along the cycle of change.

Based on where you put yourself in the change model on the previous page, what's your next move going to be?

I'm going to make a specific plan, starting with:

→ I'm moving from thinking about it to doing it. My first steps will be:

→ I'll set them up by doing these things:

→ What might get in my way is:

→ I'm becoming consistent and building habits. My bigger picture goals are:

→ I'm in the maintenance zone. I'm doing it, I just need to keep going. When I need to dig deep into my self-belief, I'll tell myself this:

→ I'll remind myself that my Big Why is:

→ I've fallen off the wagon and I need to jump back on and get back on track. I'm going to commit to these first steps today.

Go to www.helenmortonnutrition.com/resources/how-to-create-lasting-change/ to get PDF pages (The Plan, part 2) that you can fill in, or use a notepad.

Taming the mind monkeys

As you've just learned, because of the design of your brain and its nature, change is never straightforward. But another spanner in the works is your mindset. This, alongside understanding some of the neuroscience of change, are the biggest factors in whether or not we achieve our goals and sustain self-improvement.

Mindset isn't the same as willpower (we've got a section on that coming up). It's tuning into and understanding yourself and your inner world of thoughts, before making choices about how you're perceiving the things that are getting in your way and what you can try to do about them.

After all, what if there's part of you that thinks the goals or new habits you're trying to create actually *are* a threat you need saving from? What if, deep down, you don't think you'll be able to achieve them? What if there's a fear that you'll try and fail (and that this would be unacceptable or far too uncomfortable to consider)? Or a fear of what people will think if you put yourself out there and look foolish?

So much of what holds us back and prevents us from achieving and sustaining change and reaching our goals is what's going on in our minds. Fear. Self-doubt. Lack of confidence. Worry about judgement from others. Feeling vulnerable. Feeling self-conscious. Your inner critic. A belief that it's not OK to get things wrong or make mistakes. Wanting to be in control or to do things perfectly. A belief of not being good enough. Even a fear of success and what that would mean can get in the way of a healthy mindset. These are the things that whirl around in our minds and create the inner dialogue and beliefs that can sabotage our attempts to make changes and push ourselves out of our comfort zone.

One of my CBT clients calls them her mind monkeys.

If you want to achieve your goals, you need a strong mindset, and you need to learn how to counter or tame those mind monkeys!

We humans are storytellers. We create narratives and tell ourselves stories about what we think is going on. It's back to that idea of the brain wanting to know what's happening and desiring predictable outcomes. We fill in the blanks and create stories. Where your brain is designed to keep you safe and wants to predict outcomes, your mind fills in the details. It gives colour and a narrative to your experiences and your automatic responses.

When the outcome in any given situation is unclear, your mind runs through various possibilities. Because we're hardwired for safety, we have an inbuilt tendency to latch onto the outcomes that feel risky. This creates a negative bias in our minds, which means we pay more attention to worst-case scenario outcomes and skip other, tamer options.

In some instances, this works well. After all, we want an inbuilt safety valve: it stops us from doing things impulsively. It helps us to assess risk and heed warnings. This can be true in a seemingly tame situation like running, too. For example, it's important to pay attention to the signals that could lead to injury. But most of the time, in our modern world, our safety mechanisms are misfiring. We're seeing risk where there isn't any, and more often than not, we're attributing risk and holding ourselves back from a fear of being embarrassed, judged or of failing (or how we perceive failing to be).

As well as being risk averse, us humans are designed to be pack animals. We're social creatures, and part of how we've developed (and part of our original survival strategies) is by having a strong desire to be accepted and liked. So, fear of judgement from others or an intense dislike of being embarrassed can feel as risky as something with a real physical danger attached to it.

You can use this to your advantage. One of the most powerful motivators in reaching goals is to make yourself accountable to others. Train with other people. Get yourself an accountability buddy. Vocalise your goals to friends and family. You'll greatly increase the likelihood of following through on your intentions when you do.

In order to make sense of the world around us, we constantly create internal dialogues. Most of this is done subconsciously, without us even being aware of it. The rest is happening mainly automatically, without a conscious awareness of the thoughts, images and beliefs that are pinging around up there. It's estimated that we have between 60,000 and 80,000 thoughts in a day. That's 2,500 to 3,300 thoughts per hour, or up to 55 thoughts per minute. There's no way you can keep track of all of them.

Most of your thoughts never make it into your conscious awareness. But that doesn't mean they're not having an impact. That's why it's so helpful to understand how your brain works and to be mindful of the automatic triggers that drive emotions and behaviours. Then when the cues come up, such as fear or avoidance, or a strong emotional reaction, you can choose to bring awareness to them.

The thoughts that do make it into your conscious mind are often the ones linked with strong emotions or that have a perceived risk attached to them. For example, situations out of your comfort zone, or ones where you feel vulnerable to exposing yourself as not good enough.

You're likely to hook into these and let them spiral. Most of us do, until, that is, we bring conscious self-awareness to them and start to separate ourselves from our thoughts and emotions.

But how do you develop self-awareness and start tuning into your inner chatter and beliefs? And how can you start challenging your mind monkeys and get them out of the driving seat of your head?

Here's how the cognitive behavioural therapy approach to thoughts, emotions and behaviours works:

Situation:
Training for a marathon when the runs get longer.

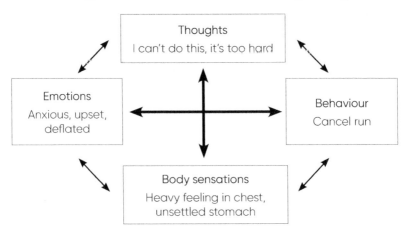

Automatic loops can generate in our minds. A situation will trigger a thought. That thought can trigger an emotion and a behaviour. Those automatic brain responses will get triggered, too, and the experience or emotion will show up as a physical sensation. They're all interconnected and are influencing one another. What you tell yourself creates emotions. An emotion can elicit a thought. A situation can be hooked into a belief about what will happen, driving you to take a certain course of action. What you do and the outcomes determine what you think. It goes round and round in a confusing, multi-directional cycle.

Most of the time, they're happening automatically. You can't always stop them, but you can become aware of your responses and start to see them for what they are: automatic reactions and nothing more than that.

Thoughts and emotions are information, not fact

Watch out for the stories you're telling yourself, especially when you're holding yourself back from going for your goals or have stopped consistently taking action to build the habits you need in order to succeed. Chances are, it's your mindset getting in the way.

"If you change the way you look at things, the things you look at change." - Wayne Dyer

One summer, not so long ago, I was running on Hampstead Heath in London, near where I live. I was enjoying my run and feeling in a flow with it. I ran past two people out walking and one of them started laughing. In my rational head, I knew that it was unlikely they were laughing at me. The Heath is full of runners and there's nothing that makes me particularly stand out when I join the throng, but I automatically reacted as if they were. I felt a flash of shame and embarrassment and my flow was disrupted. I momentarily slowed down my pace and started to feel heavy and ungainly. I had to consciously change these reactions to get back into my stride.

I knew enough to spot what was happening, but, even then, it still affected me and what I was doing. I eventually got my flow back, but if that had happened years ago, when I'd just started running and felt awkward and self-conscious (and held a belief that I couldn't run and didn't belong in that world), it could have been a huge setback. For some people, it could have been enough to prevent them from going back out running.

A week later and I was out on the Heath again. This time, as I ran past a group of people, one of them called out to their friend, "Go, you!" Again, I knew they weren't saying it to me, but even so I noticed myself responding to it. I got a spring in my step, my pace picked up, my posture improved and my shoulders went back. I held my head up higher and I felt more confident. All from a fleeting reaction to a passing comment that wasn't even made about me. (Incidentally, I left this one to carry on playing out and just enjoyed the impact.)

The internalisations and interpretations that we create have real impact. What we respond to, what we go on to say in our inner dialogue and what we believe about situations and ourselves all matter. We can choose to let them play out unchecked, knowing that they have such a powerful influence, or we can start to shine a spotlight on them and bring some curious observation into the mix. Your job with your mindset is to notice the patterns that come up and get you thinking, feeling or acting in unhelpful ways that take you off course and away from your goals. Then you can start to disrupt the cycle.

Compare the first diagram to the one over the page.

What you say to yourself *really* matters

Your self-talk has a direct impact on how you feel. So does what you do: your actions send out a message loud and clear about what you think is going on in any given situation. If you avoid doing something because you're unsure or afraid, you reinforce the belief that there's something to avoid. If you only ever go so far in your new habits, you show yourself that you can't go any further, and that becomes your pattern.

Situation:

Training for a marathon when the runs get longer.

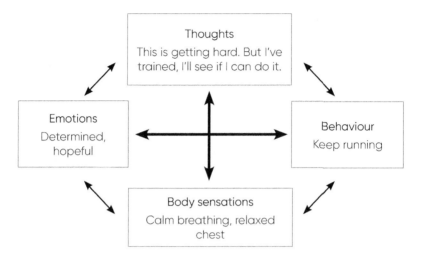

In order to move past any limiting beliefs about what you can achieve, tune in and start noticing your thoughts, emotions and typical responses. Then you can either sit with them or change them. Either way, what you're not going to do is let your thoughts and emotions dictate your actions. If you don't change this bit, you're never going to show yourself just what you're capable of.

> If you don't believe in yourself and see your goals as possible, you're never going to go the distance.

Ways to spot your mind monkeys at play

* When you get stuck or feel a block around what you think you're capable of, tune into your body. What's coming up? Where are you holding your emotions? What sensations do you notice?

* When you find yourself avoiding something, feeling unsure or slipping back into old habits, dial into your inner chatter.

* Write down what you're saying to yourself.

* Watch out for that inner critic. Are you talking down to yourself?

* Are you feeling frustrated that you can't seem to get past a certain point? Ask yourself why.

* Sit and reflect. Be in silence with your thoughts and see what comes up.

* Notice any patterns of behaviour when you don't follow through on your goals, and be honest with yourself. Are you avoiding or procrastinating?

* Ask yourself how it feels to put yourself out there and do something challenging.

* Examine the messages you've received throughout your life around making mistakes or failing.

* Tune into any beliefs you've been holding about not being able to do something or not being good enough.

* As you move out of your comfort zone, notice if you have images or mini movies playing out in your mind about the things that feel uncomfortable or intense.

Once you've started bringing some awareness to your thoughts and emotions, the next step is to look at how accurate they are.

All of us have something called thought distortions. They're skewed ways of thinking, and if we don't stop to question them, they'll lead us along narratives and patterns that aren't usually helpful. They'll reinforce those loops and keep you stuck in perspectives that aren't always true or useful.

Some examples of thought distortions that can get in your way:

- → All-or-nothing thinking.
- → Believing you're not good enough to do something.
- → Believing you'll fail before you've even tried.
- → Thinking you need to be naturally good at something in order to do it.
- → Needing things to be perfect.
- → Believing you have to be an expert in order to participate.
- → Having narrow definitions of success and achievement.
- → Catastrophising.
- → Fear of failure.
- → Seeing mistakes as failures.
- → Mind reading, thinking others are judging you.
- → Holding limiting self-beliefs.
- → Holding yourself up to unattainably high standards.
- → Believing you can't change so never getting started.

These are just some of the inaccurate ways we can think about ourselves and the world around us. Start tuning into the thoughts and beliefs in your mind and you'll uncover all sorts of stories that you're telling yourself.

Once you've started noticing the patterns and skewed ways of thinking playing out, you can start to question them. You can reflect on whether or not they're really true. How likely is it that what you're believing will happen? What would you do if it did? What's another way of looking at things? You can open up your perspective and change the way you're feeling or perceiving the situation. You can choose what you're going to do. It puts you back in the driving seat.

Fear = a belief something bad will happen + a lack of confidence in your ability to cope.

A big part of the limiting beliefs that hold us back is the fear of something bad happening, and that we won't be able to cope. We all know what this feels like. Have you ever avoided doing something because you feared you might not actually be able to do it and would be exposed as not good enough? Have you ever procrastinated because you were worried about making mistakes or about what others would think about you? Have you ever not gone after what you truly wanted because of a fear of being judged or making a fool of yourself?

Letting your limiting beliefs determine what you do keeps you stuck in the loop of feeling that you're not capable, so you never get to show yourself a different outcome. You keep the story going and each time you procrastinate, avoid, give up or talk down to yourself, you reinforce that story and strengthen your belief in it.

The release and mindset growth comes when you do things despite your fears or reservations. You give yourself the opportunity to see that:

a. Either the bad thing hasn't happened (or isn't as bad as you thought it would be).

b. You can handle it.

You give yourself the opportunity to see how capable you actually are, or the opportunity to build your skills if you need to progress.

When you learn this, there's freedom in trying new things and working towards your goals, even when you're not sure what's going to happen.

If you want to start moving past your limiting beliefs and changing your internal narrative when it's not helping you, start asking yourself these questions whenever your mind monkeys show up.

→ What's the story I'm telling myself?

→ How do I know it's true?

→ What evidence do I have that it's true?

→ What evidence do I have that it's not true?

→ What's the worst that could happen?

→ How would I cope if it did?

→ Has this happened before?

→ What's another possible way of looking at this?

→ Are there any thought distortions at play?

→ What's one thing I can do to help myself right now?

A final question to ask yourself when you're finding it hard to keep on track with your goals is this:

→ Is your desire to try stronger than your fear of failing?

Test out taking the answers you come up with to the above questions and turning them into snappy mantras to say to yourself when you're feeling unsure or finding it hard to reach your goals. A good mantra will have an instant impact on the way you're feeling and open up your perspective on the beliefs you're holding in that moment.

Flexing the willpower muscle

"Discipline is choosing what you want most over what you want now."- Shaa Wasmund MBE

The last thing we're going to look at in this chapter on creating a mindset that helps not hinders is willpower.

Willpower is simply the building of discipline regarding where you put your focus and attention. It's not an innate quality that you either have or don't have. You can learn it and build on it. It's the discipline of choosing what you want most over what you want in this moment.

A large part of creating consistent habits and changing behaviours in the long-term comes down to what we call willpower. We too often talk about having willpower or not, as if it's something outside of our control that we're powerless to do anything about. How many times have you heard someone say (or said it yourself) that they just didn't have the willpower to resist a temptation or to keep going with a new habit or routine?

Let's change the script on this.

Your bed might seem super comfy and enticing when your alarm goes off for a 6am run and it's raining outside. It's these moments when we dig deep and choose what we want bigger-picture wise: our ultimate goal over our preference in the moment? Our Big Why over a temporary pleasure?

This is why setting up your routines and regular practices well is so important. Train your willpower: if your run is mapped out, your trainers are by the door, your running kit is out ready for you to put on and you've played it all out in your mind already, you're making it much easier to create willpower.

Tell yourself you choose the 6am run because it will get you closer to your goal. Tune in to what you find enjoyable about it. Bring self-awareness to the process of your brain trying to talk you out of it and steer you back to what feels comfortable and safe. Notice the stories you're telling yourself about whether or not you can do it.

Willpower isn't a magical quality that's outside of your construct. You can develop your willpower just like anything else. It's about choices and where you place your focus and attention when your motivation starts to fade.

If you tell yourself that you just don't have the willpower, it's like telling yourself it's game over. There's nothing you can do, right? You're not self-disciplined enough. Tell yourself this and your mind monkeys will have a field day. You'll let your thoughts spiral off into all sorts of negative beliefs about yourself and how you never see things through or just don't have the skills or talent.

This brings you down and serves to demotivate you. Surely, you're not going to carry on trying to do something when you're clearly failing at it?

Instead, try looking at willpower as something you can build. A muscle you can flex. Choose where you put your focus and attention, because that's all willpower really is – making a choice to take action on what you want the most, rather than what you want in this moment.

Show yourself that you can commit to seeing things through when you put your mind to it. Build your willpower muscle through daily activities, and use these to create a strong sense of identity as someone who finishes things. This can be as simple as making your bed when you get up in the morning. See tasks through to the end when you start them. Finish the action. When you do this, you'll be building your willpower and self-discipline. After all, how you do one thing is how you do all things, When you then want to apply willpower to your fitness goals or training, you've already got a blueprint for knowing that you've got the ability to follow through and complete something.

Ways to build willpower:

→ Practise actively focusing on your day-to-day activities.

→ Increase your focus and attention by being more mindful in the moment.

→ Show yourself that you do complete what you set out to do. Do this with your bigger goals, as well as with your small, day-to-day ones.

→ Make choices today that your future self will thank you for. (Practise visualising yourself in the future, and relate the choices and actions you make today to how they'll form the person you'll become.)

→ Ask yourself how you'll feel at the end of the day when you're about to go to bed – will you feel proud and pleased about your decisions or choices?

→ Tap into your Big Why and remind yourself what's driving you. Make choices based on this rather than what you feel tempted by in the moment.

→ Build your willpower step by step, just like you're building your habits to get you towards your goals.

So, to successfully make the changes you want in your life, keep tuning in. Keep learning about yourself. Keep being curious and questioning the story you're telling yourself, and keep going as you move towards your goals. Show yourself a different story.

THE FINAL WORD

Individuality

You have heard me say this several times already. There is no 'one-size-fits-all' answer to nutrition for female runners.

Your journey is yours, and my journey is mine.

You'll see this every time you head out of the door for a run.

Women of all ages, heights, shapes and sizes running the streets and trails. And if you were to ask every female runner you came across what they eat and drink on a typical day when they feel great and run strong, I guarantee that their answers would be different.

Some of you thrive on a gluten-free diet, some of you may eat pasta twice a day. Some of you eat loads of veggies, while some of you favour fruit. Some of you enjoy cooking, while some of you prefer ready prepared meals. None of these things are necessarily better than the other.

> The main thing is that the way YOU eat makes YOU feel great and able to smash your running goals.

When it comes to running and exercise, there are those of you who want to run longer and further each year, and many of you who are more than happy to run shorter distances consistently. Neither way is right or wrong, as it is a personal preference. You are a runner whatever speed or distance you run.

Women are not men

For a book dedicated to female runners, this is an important (if obvious) point. On the surface, men and women are the same. After all, we are all human beings. But male and female brains do not function in quite the same way. Women have reproductive organs and hormones that men do not. It could also be argued that women and men are treated differently within the running community, but that is not something I am going to get into here! But here are some differences I'm willing to share:

- ✓ Women, in general, need fewer carbohydrates than men to produce a similar intensity run.
- ✓ Women have different dietary fat requirements for health and running performance.
- ✓ Women tend to have a higher body fat percentage than men. This is not something for us to curse, it's simply the beautiful way we have been designed.
- ✓ Women's fat is stored primarily around their hips and thighs, while for men, excess body fat tends to sit centrally.
- ✓ Women tend to have less muscle and a lower metabolic rate than men.

All these facts make you amazing and very much deserving of feeding your body with exactly the right food and drink to feel full of energy and run strong.

Fuel for the work required

I love the saying, "Fuel for the work required." Basically, it means adjusting the food you eat on a day-to-day or even a meal-to-meal basis, depending on your training and life needs.

This new phrase was devised in 2016 by James P. Morton, the head of nutrition for the Team Sky cycling team, and the sports scientist Samuel G. Impey, who co-authored a study around planned, purposeful carbohydrate intake preceding training.

Getting the timing right of your food makes a massive difference to how you think, feel and run.

Each day is different. Some days you may wake feeling energised and full of life, and then sail through your work and long training run. Other days may be more of a struggle. Perhaps you have PMS, or anxiety will rear its ugly head and you will only have enough time to run a few miles.

What and when you eat on these two days should be different. Needs are different, so adjust your food and drink to accommodate this.

Eat well and run strong, ladies!

RESOURCES

Here are some contacts and information sources that you might find useful in terms of supporting your health, wellbeing and running.

BANT (British Association for Nutrition and Lifestyle Medicine): bant.org.uk/

The Institute for Optimum Nutrition (ION): www.ion.ac.uk/

myDNAhealth genetic testing: mydnahealth.co.uk/

BEAT eating disorders charity: www.beateatingdisorders.org.uk/

MIND for better mental health: www.mind.org.uk/

Urine colour chart: www.nhsinform.scot/campaigns/hydration

England Athletics, where you can find your local running club: www.englandathletics.org/find-an-athletics-club/

ACKNOWLEDGEMENTS

I want to start by thanking all of my friends who have run, chatted, laughed and cried with me for so many miles over the years.

Kirsten, all the running we did when the girls were little was the best antidote to the early challenges of motherhood, and I hope we can run together again one day.

Marissa, you have been my rock forever and I can't thank you enough for all of your unconditional support and encouragement, plus, of course, for joining me on many epic runs in extreme temperatures.

Steph, our weekly runs training for your first half got me through a very difficult period of my life, and I am so happy that we are running together again now. Perhaps one day we will better our Charterhouse 3rd place finish!

Helen, I was so lucky to have met you at the start of my first Fox Ultra. Your advice and encouragement were invaluable, and you made the experience so much fun.

Elaine, it has been brilliant running with you over the last few years, and I cannot thank you enough for hauling me up Chinthurst Hill, both before and after my foot surgery.

Nikki, the runs and walks we did together, once I was given the go ahead to run again, were invaluable, and you are a constant source of inspiration to me.

Thanks must also go to Emily and the Gentle and Successful Leadership group for kindly pushing me forward to get on with writing, and for making this book specific to female runners. A special thank you to Lara for motivating me every step of the way. I could not have done this without you.

Also, thank you to Jackie for all your ideas on the cover design aspects of the book, and Adriana for your unwavering faith in me.

A huge thank you to Eve and Clare for believing in me and the book, and for spending so much of your free time writing. I am so pleased and proud that you both decided to come on board. Clare, your Mindworks group is awesome, and I hope this book inspires others to dream big and achieve their goals. Eve, it feels like a lifetime ago that we started studying at ION; you have achieved so much since then and I know you will continue to do so.

Finally, of course, thanks to Alexa for backing me on this project and for being fundamental in getting my book out of my head and onto paper.

Keep on running, ladies!

Printed in Great Britain
by Amazon

32730811R00126